Organ Transplants

Organ Transplants

THE MORAL ISSUES

by
Catherine Lyons

THE WESTMINSTER PRESS
Philadelphia

Copyright © MCMLXX The Westminster Press

ISBN 0-664-24897-7

LIBRARY OF CONGRESS CATALOG CARD No. 70-120139

BOOK DESIGN BY
DOROTHY ALDEN SMITH

Published by The Westminster Press®
Philadelphia, Pennsylvania

PRINTED IN THE UNITED STATES OF AMERICA

Contents

ACKNOWLEDGMENTS   9

INTRODUCTION   11

I HUMAN EXPERIMENTATION
    AND ORGAN TRANSPLANTATION   24

        Medicine in Dialogue
        Human Experimentation in General
        The Experimental Nature
            of Organ Transplantation

II MEDICINE'S QUEST TO REDEFINE DEATH   48

        An Irony of Medical Advance
        The Process of Dying
        Three Approaches to a Redefinition
        Redefining Death: The Moral Issue

III THE GIFT OF LIFE (ORGAN PROCUREMENT:
     RECIPIENT SELECTION)   75

        Dawn of a New Day and Its Limitations
        The Problem of Organ Procurement
        Recipient Selection

IV ORGAN TRANSPLANTATION:
        RETROSPECT AND PROSPECT   109
            The Shape of Tomorrow
            Looking Back
            Looking Forward

APPENDIX: UNIFORM ANATOMICAL GIFT ACT   119

NOTES   127

SELECTED BIBLIOGRAPHY   131

Acknowledgments

My heartfelt thanks to Dr. Henry E. Kolbe, adviser, pastor, and personal friend, whose sensitivity to and understanding of the problems that arise in writing and in preparing a manuscript for publication have enabled me to finish this work. His critical mind and gentle manner have contributed to this writing and to my own way of thinking in more ways than I can express in words. His clarity of thought and ability to discern the central issues of the questions with which I was dealing opened for me those doors of understanding which are essential to any thorough evaluation of ethical problems.

My sincere appreciation to my father and my brother, the Doctors Alexander J. and Russell A. Lyons, for the assistance they have given me in securing research material. My thanks to Miss Marsha Barron for her help in organizing the bibliography, and to Dr. Wolfgang Roth, of Garrett Theological Seminary, and Paul Blanton, of Northwestern Uni-

versity, for their time and helpful comments. My
sincere thanks to Mrs. Monica LaVeille, who, on but
a moment's notice, accepted the responsibility for
typing the final draft of the manuscript.

Finally, my deep gratitude to Vera and Russ Watts,
who graciously opened their home to me during the
crucial final weeks of writing on the thesis from
which this book has developed. I am deeply grateful
to Miss Carol Jennings, whose enthusiastic support
for the entire writing project kept me going at those
times when my own enthusiasm had burned low.

Introduction

On Saturday, December 3, 1967, at the Groote
Schuur Hospital, Cape Town, South Africa, an ordi-
nary organ was used in an extraordinary event. Dr.
Christiaan Barnard transplanted the heart of Denise
Ann Darvall into the chest of Louis Washkansky. The
operation was a surgical success and another first in
medical history. Transplants of other organs had pre-
dated this occasion, but for various reasons this was
the special event.

Prior to this, fathers had donated kidneys to their
children, brothers and sisters had donated their kidneys to one another—but here was something different. An organ from the dead was used to sustain
the dying: from the dead there came life, and one's
misfortune became another's hope. The difference
between these two situations is simple. A man has
two kidneys. He can give up one and live. But a man
has only one heart. The death of one person is pre-

requisite to the life of another in heart transplantations.

December 3, 1967, marked the beginning of a new
era: the era of heart transplantations. Few people
interested in recent medical advances can reflect on
that day without bowing their heads in awe and
wonder. And yet, more than awe and wonder surrounded that day. The legal and ethical problems
that have arisen as a result of recent medical advances are enough to stagger the imagination.

How medical science is to overcome its moral
dilemmas is yet to be seen. If the present situation
is a portent of the future, however, medical scientists
will not make their decisions in a vacuum. Philoso-
phers, theologians, lawyers, and doctors have already
joined in dialogue. There are certain decisions that
medicine in the end will have to make for itself, but
in the final analysis it will be seen that philosophy,
theology, and law will have played an integral part
in the decision-making process. Such dialogue is
necessary because the subject matter with which
medical science deals does not lend itself to easy
decisions in the area of ethics. Medical scientists deal
in empirical data. They make decisions by weighing
the measurable. And yet, many of the decisions that
must be made now are those involving value judgments.

As medical science stands on the threshold of even
more astounding scientific and technological break-
throughs, it must come to grips with itself in an effort
to see what implications its past achievements have

had on the present and what its present capabilities hold in store for the future.

Recent scientific and technological developments have made human organ transplantation an accomplished fact. For all of this, man stands today where men for ages have stood: pondering the meaning of life and of death. Medical science is able to initiate life in a test tube. It can speak of the chemical formulation and the biological structure of life, but on the meaning of life medical science falls silent. This is one dilemma of the present situation. With the need to remove certain vital organs from cadavers as soon as possible after the death of the person, medical science is pushed to question what constitutes death. Unable to comprehend the meaning of life and of death, medical scientists are left to define what constitutes death and to establish a set of criteria by which death may be determined.

Death has been defined traditionally as the "permanent cessation of spontaneous heart beat and respiration."[1] Medical science, however, has rendered this definition almost meaningless because of the development and perfection of artificial sustainers, such as the respirator and the cardiac pacemaker. Vital bodily functions, the cessation of which once constituted the criteria of death, may now be prolonged almost indefinitely by the use of artificial means. In many instances, that cessation of bodily functions which once denoted death may be avoided. The physician's ability to prolong life has complicated the task of defining death.

In this age of seemingly unlimited possibilities, medical science finds itself caught in the question of the "is" and the "ought." The fact that certain things can be done is not justification in itself that they ought to be done. Sir Theodore Fox cautions medical scientists on this point. "We shall have to refrain from doing things merely because we know how to do them."[2] Recent medical advances have put us in a moral quandary. Does the fact that medical science knows how to prolong life justify the transgression of a man's right to die with dignity when there is no hope of recovery? The question of the "is" and the "ought" merits serious moral consideration lest the extraordinary become the conventional and we succumb to the "temptation to subordinate the person to the technique."[3]

As medicine increases its scientific and technological knowledge, there arises an ever-pressing need to realize that knowledge, like physical power, must be held in check. Knowledge, like physical power that goes unchecked, has the potential of being a highly destructive force.

By "holding in check" is not meant the "limiting of knowledge." What is meant is checking the utilization of knowledge when such utilization of facts and data would be destructive of human well-being. This is analogous to the holding in check of physical power. To hold a man's physical power in check does not mean prohibiting him from developing his muscularity beyond a certain point, but it means holding in check how he utilizes his muscularity or physical power. There is nothing morally reprehensible about a strong body, but how a man uses his physical power may be morally reprehensible if he uses it in a manner destructive of his or another's well-being. The same holds true in medicine.

This is again the question of the "is" and the "ought." Physicians ought not always do all that they are able to do any more than a man with superior physical strength ought always to do all that he is able to do. A quick review of the history of civilization reminds one that the utilization of man's knowledge and his physical power has not always had at its core respect for the human being.

Respect for the human being (or human well-being) must always be the check between medical knowledge and the utilization of its facts and data in overt action. Upon the establishment of "respect for the human being" as the criterion of any action, another moral dilemma arises. This is so because there are no absolutes to tell one what "respect for the human being" means in every case. In one case it may call for the resuscitation of a person; in another case it may call for the failure to do so. In one case it may call for the transplantation of a heart; in another case it may call for the refusal to use such extraordinary measures. Respect for the human being requires that we see life to be more than brain function, heartbeat, and respiration. It requires that we think in terms of quality of life rather than in terms of physiological life signs.

Medicine is thus faced with the task of questioning

whether it ought always to do what it is technically
and scientifically capable of doing. The burden of this
question cannot be shifted from the shoulders of the
doctor onto the shoulders of the philosopher. The
philosopher and the theologian may (and must) join
in dialogue with the physician, but the physician
himself must wrestle with the question and take himself to task on the issue. The question of the "is" and
the "ought" demands that the doctor be responsible
in utilizing his knowledge in overt actions. At times,
the question of the "is" and the "ought," in keeping
with the criterion of respect for human well-being,
will demand that the doctor be responsible enough
not to do all that he is capable of doing.

This criterion of respect for human well-being or
for the human being not only must guide medicine in
the utilization of its knowledge in overt actions, it
must guide it in its acquisition of knowledge.

Valuable knowledge has been gained through
human experimentation, but human experimentation
for the sake of pure knowledge is morally questionable. Medicine deals in scientific knowledge and
technique. These are the tools of its trade. But scientific knowledge and technique are not its end. The
end of medicine is to promote human well-being.
Scientific knowledge and technique are means of
attaining this end. Human experimentation for the
sake of pure knowledge is morally questionable in
that knowledge becomes the goal or the end and man
becomes the means only. Immanuel Kant's practical
imperative addresses this issue. "Act so that you treat

humanity, whether in your own person or in that of another, always as an end and never as a means only. ... Man ... is not a thing, and thus not something to be used merely as a means; he must always be regarded in all his actions as an end in himself."[4]

Knowledge must be respectful of the human being. This is true whether it is knowledge already gained and wanting for utilization or knowledge on the horizon and yet to be had. It is the responsibility of medical science to see that knowledge in its utilization and its acquisition is respectful of man.

Some will say, no doubt, that this is much to ask of medical science, and much it is to ask, but not too much. Much is asked and will be asked of a science that has at its disposal techniques and instruments for the promotion or destruction of human well-being.

If medical science stands on the threshold of the unknown, it also stands on the brink of an age demanding a technology within the limits of morality. In stressing that the end of medicine is to promote human well-being, issue is being taken against the traditional idea that the purpose of medicine is the prolongation of life. A twofold problem has arisen around the prolongation of life as the purpose of medicine. First, this is an age of technological genius in which life may be prolonged indefinitely. Second, just what it is that constitutes life is open to question.

These two problems merit individual consideration. With regard to the first problem, it is important to note that modern technology has provided medical science with a number of lifesaving devices. Among

these are the resuscitator and the cardiac pacemaker.
In that these devices save a life, they also prolong a
life. But it is true that they may, in fact, prolong a life
without saving that life in another quite meaningful
sense of "life."

By the phrase "saving a life," or the word "lifesaving," we mean a change for the better, where a
person is rescued or delivered in a moment of peril
from a life-endangering situation. In saving a drowning child, a man literally pulls the child out of his
moment of peril and the child's life is saved or, so to
speak, spared. In that the child's life is saved or
spared, it is prolonged. This idea of saving a life
carries with it the connotation that the person whose
life has been saved will be able to go on to live that
life of his own accord.

Within the realm of medical science, the resuscitator, the cardiac pacemaker, and new surgical techniques have served the same purpose as the man who
came across the drowning child. They have pulled
people out of their moments of peril, saved their lives,
and sent them on their way to live their lives. Each
day a lucky few are saved by means of organ transplantations. Dr. Philip Blaiberg was an example of a
person whose life had been saved through an organ
transplantation. What qualifies that event in Cape
Town as a lifesaving event is that Blaiberg was
enabled to go on of his own accord to live his life.
But what if Blaiberg's life after surgery had depended
upon artificial means, such as the resuscitator? Might
one not hesitate to say that his life had been saved?

If his life had depended upon artificial sustainers, it would be more correct to say that his life was being prolonged. The point being made here is that of saving a life versus the mere prolongation of that life. Saving a life necessarily implies the prolongation of that life. The fact that a life is being prolonged, however, does not necessarily imply that that life has been saved.

The prolongation of life, as the purpose of medicine, in an age in which a life may be prolonged without there being any hope for the person's recovery, becomes morally questionable. The prolongation of life as the purpose of medicine was feasible in an age in which the prolongation of life and the saving of life were virtually synonymous. And no doubt there was a time prior to this age of technological genius when no life was prolonged that was not, in fact, saved. This would have been so because in the absence of artificial sustainers a man would have been enabled to go on to live his life of his own accord or he would have died.

That age of medicine, prior to this age of artificial sustainers, was truly an age of "life or death." This is not the case today, however. It is more correct to call this the age of "life, death, and mere prolongation," with death, all too often, being permitted only after a long-fought battle to die on the part of the patient. To use the poignant words of Dr. G. E. Schreiner, professor of medicine at Georgetown University, we are in an age in which we must decide "how many ribs to break with cardiac massage, or how many old

people should unnecessarily be subjected to thousands of dollars' worth of resuscitation, or whether it
is ever possible to die without a series of cardiac
arrests."[5]

Dr. Schreiner's witty statement underlies a serious
moral dilemma: the prolongation of life where there
is no hope of recovery (that is to say, where the life
cannot be saved). Whereas the resuscitator and the
cardiac pacemaker and numerous other artificial devices have been instrumental in saving lives, they
have also been used in the mere prolongation of life
when, because of the extent and seriousness of the
illness, the person's hope and future were already
dead. The moral reprehensibility of such an action is
to be seen in that, in not being able to save the
person's life on the one hand and in not permitting
the person to die on the other, such devices actually
confine the person to his perilous situation. He becomes a prisoner, so to speak, who has been sen-
tenced neither to life nor to death but to mere
existence devoid of future. Whatever else this may
be, it is not respect for human well-being. Respect
for human well-being has to do with life and the
living of it. And when there is no life to live, it has to
do with permitting the person to die.

Today, when medical science can prolong life indefinitely without enabling the person to live life on
his own, there is the need to rethink what the purpose
of medicine should be. Medical science is strong in
knowledge and yet it lacks the wisdom of the sage

who knew that just as a man is born so he shall also die. Medical science needs the wisdom of the sage for guidance, for to have knowledge is not to be wise, and to gain in knowledge is not to negate the need to be guided by wisdom.

The mere prolongation of life stands at odds with the idea of the promotion of human well-being. No matter how one looks at it, there is no well-being in a life that is endlessly prolonged without hope. There is only the agony and the suffering, be it physical or psychological, of not being able to live on the one hand and not being permitted to die on the other. The promotion of human well-being has not only to do with life but with the quality of that life. The person's well-being, rather than the quantity of years, is the determining factor.

The second problem arising around the prolongation of life as the purpose of medicine is that the life which is being prolonged is not necessarily human life. Medical science is cautious not to violate life. But in its caution against violating life, it is apt to violate the authentic human dimension of life. Vegetation is life just as human life is life. Yet vegetation is not human life. Man's possession of a brain sets him apart from vegetable life. Man's capacity to reason with his brain sets him apart from animal life. Human life depends upon a brain that endows man with the capacity to reason. This is to say that, in man, when the brain is dead human life is dead. This is so even though there remains cellular and biological life. In the face of brain death, the body vegetates. It lives like a vegetable: inactive, passive, and unthinking.

With the prolongation of life as its purpose, time and again medical science has found itself in the hideous position of sustaining a mindless body. In resuscitating such a body the biological activities of the organs are sustained, but human life is neither retained nor regained. Such a situation is analogous, not to the candle that has been blown out and can be relighted, but to the candle whose wick, having burned down or otherwise been destroyed, has lost its source of activity and that which gave it its distinction of having been a candle.

With its present technological skill, and the prolongation of life as its purpose, medical science finds itself in a dilemma: that of being able to prolong life without necessarily being able to save that life and that of the prolongation of life that is not necessarily human life.

The promotion of human well-being must be not only the purpose of medicine but the criterion for the utilization and acquisition of scientific and technological knowledge. What concrete actions afford the promotion of human well-being cannot be decided outside the actual situation. The promotion of human well-being as the purpose of medicine is, at the same time, medicine's dilemma. With regard to the promotion of human well-being one thing can be said for sure: only they will know what it means who are sensitive to what it is that constitutes human life.

If medicine is entrusted with a mission, it is the mission of healing the sick and relieving suffering. Those whom it holds in its care are the injured, the sick, and the dying. In such an arena there is no room for depersonalizing or dehumanizing forces. Medicine must seek the wisdom to know where it is going with the decisions it makes. The danger that is implicit today is that of subordinating the person to the technique. In the midst of its technological advances, medical science must be cautious lest its intimate concern for the sick and the dying be pushed aside by its passion for knowledge. In medicine it is not the pessimist who writes that haste makes waste. Rather, it is the optimist who knows both that success is possible and that the way to success is often a painstakingly slow journey.

Human Experimentation
and Organ Transplantation

MEDICINE IN DIALOGUE

The practice of medicine involves a dialogue between persons. This dialogue takes place at various levels. At one level it involves the physicians themselves and those who aid them in their task. The physician stands in constant dialogue with the present through his dialogue with other physicians, while at the same time he maintains a dialogue with the past and the future. To be in dialogue with the past and with the future is to review the accomplishments and failures of the past and to question what lies in the future as a result of the past and of the present. The physician who is in dialogue with the present is serving the time by maintaining the tension between past accomplishments and future capabilities. Such dialogue between medicine's past and its future is integral to scientific progress. But such dialogue does not constitute the whole of medicine in dialogue.

Fundamentally, the practice of medicine is involved in a dialogue between those engaged in the science of healing and those who seek relief from their sufferings. At the heart of such dialogue must lie a very personal concern for the promotion of human well-being.

Being in dialogue involves listening and responding. It involves the initiative to join in relating to another being. Dialogue involves relationship. The dialogue carried on between the doctor and the patient is dependent upon the doctor-patient relationship. The sick or injured person indicates his desire to initiate a relationship through his plea to be relieved of his suffering. The relationship is actualized when the physician, acknowledging the person's plea, enters into relationship with him in an effort to achieve his (the patient's) end. The dialogue that takes place must be, on the part of the doctor, one of being aware of and responding to the need of the other.

There are certain moral considerations that must enter into any relationship that is based upon the need of a person to be made well or whole again. Three considerations basic to such a relationship are trust, honesty, and respect for human well-being. When these three considerations are present within the relationship the door is held open for dialogue while at the same time barriers are built to guard against the misuse of humanity.

Trust and honesty are to a large extent dependent upon each other. This is to be seen by the fact that a person often hesitates to be completely honest with someone he does not trust, feeling that one ought to be worthy of another's honesty. On the other hand, one hesitates to trust someone who is not honest.

In order for a patient to trust a doctor, the patient must in some way find assurance that the doctor always has the patient's well-being as his prime concern. It is, therefore, the responsibility of the physician to have the patient's well-being as his goal. This is a serious responsibility, and it is made even more serious by the fact that the sick or injured person is both the subject and the object of medical science. He is the subject for whom medical science exists and the object through whom it gains much of its knowledge. It should be noted, however, that the aspect of the relationship in which the patient stands as the object of medical science cannot be avoided. This is so because anything the doctor does to the patient will in some way increase his knowledge, if only by reaffirming some piece of knowledge he gained in a past similar experience. What can and must be avoided, however, is that situation in which man becomes merely the object of medical science.

Since dialogue between the doctor and the patient stands at the heart of the practice of medicine, any scientific experiment that destroys or puts the doctor-patient relationship and dialogue in jeopardy is morally questionable.

Much criticism and many questions have arisen today around the so-called experimental nature of recent organ transplantations. Such criticism surrounds the fear that man may become merely the object of scientific investigation. In the wake of such criticism, it is important to question the idea of human experimentation in general and the experimental nature of organ transplantation in particular.

HUMAN EXPERIMENTATION IN GENERAL

It is necessary to realize that any medicine, technique, or device is experimental at the outset. A perfected medicine, technique, or device is not discovered. The medicine, technique, or device itself is discovered: the perfection comes of a slow birth. It is born out of the process of trial and error: a process that is frequently tediously and painstakingly slow. The fact that something is experimental does not, in itself, make it morally questionable. What is and always must be open to question is the end one has in mind with regard to the experiment.

The question of performing experimentations on human beings comes as a dilemma to medical science. In the words of Samuel Enoch Stumpf: "The dilemma we face is how to achieve two highly desirable goals, namely, the expansion of medical knowledge and the protection of the dignity and the security of the individual."[6]

Progress in medicine depends upon medicine's increase in its scientific and technological knowledge. The knowledge of how to do is prerequisite to the doing, and the discovery of knowing how to do frequently involves the use of human beings as the means to the acquisition of that knowledge.

Medical science is intimately bound up in the task

of relieving human suffering. It should be realized that there is neither the need for medical science nor the possibility of its progress apart from man in his suffering and need.

It is as inconceivable that medical science will not use man in its acquisition of knowledge as it is that one man could exist without using other men. Using people is one dimension of our relationship with them. And using a patient for the acquisition of knowledge is one dimension of medicine's relationship with those who seek its help.

The crucial question for man and for medical science concerns the extent to which one can use people without misusing or abusing them. When does using a person become misusing a person? This is a question in ethics for which there are no easy answers. Our everyday relationships teach us that to use a person is not necessarily to do wrong to that person or to act injuriously toward him; and yet, one knows that there is a fine line between use and misuse. One can use a person too much and too often, to the point that the person is being misused simply by overuse. We also know that we misuse people when we see them as objects of our control, subject to our whims and fancies and the gratification of our desires. We misuse another person when we use him as the means to an end of which he cannot have a share, but for which he will have paid heavily in life or limb. To deceive a person is always to misuse the person. We misuse a person when we deceive him into thinking that his well-being can benefit from

what we are having him do, when we know that in
the end his well-being can in no way benefit from
the end because the end is not his to enjoy. Such
deceit is misuse, and this is one reason why honesty,
as a moral consideration, is necessary in the doctor-
patient relationship.

One can use a person and still maintain a relationship of love and respect for him. Love and respect
for man stand at odds with the misuse of man. To
have love and respect for a person is to see him as a
human being with certain rights and privileges,
among them that of being treated as a human being.
To love and respect a person does not mean that one
will never use him, for in loving and respecting him
we also know that we are dependent upon him. When
my car breaks down, I am dependent upon another
person to get me to the airport, just as in my moments
of weakness I am dependent upon the strength of
another person. I use that person and his strength
as a means to my own strength. To be so dependent
upon that other person and his strength is to use
him, but it is not necessarily to misuse him. We
spend our lives in dependence on others and in use
of others.

Dependency and use are virtually correlative, but
dependency and misuse are not correlative. Medical
science, therefore, has neither the right nor the moral
justification to misuse people any more than one man
has the right or the moral justification to misuse
another man.

The medical scientist's misuse of man is not differ-

ent from man's misuse of man in general. For example, to make a showpiece out of a patient is to deny
that patient his human dignity and his right of pri-
vacy. In such a case the patient is misused through
overuse. In addition, medical science misuses a patient when it leads him to believe that the knowledge
it can gain through using him as an experimental
subject will benefit him when it knows that because
of the critical nature of his condition there is no
such thing as hope or benefit for him. Likewise, the
patient is misused when he is used as a means to an
end in which he can share but for which he unknow-
ingly will pay a disproportionate amount in his own
well-being.

It is not fiction but fact that people are misused
in these ways each day. Man is always vulnerable
to misuse, and he is especially vulnerable to such
misuse through human experimentation when the
acquisition of knowledge is seen to be of the utmost
importance. For this reason it is the moral obligation
of medical science to establish safeguards whereby
in using man as a means to the acquisition of knowledge man will not be a victim of misuse.

To prevent unethical experimentation, Dr. H. K.
Beecher suggests two safeguards: "First, there should
be . . . informed consent; secondly, 'there is the
more reliable safeguard provided by the presence
of an intelligent, informed, conscientious, compassionate, responsible investigator.' "[7] The first safeguard that Dr. Beecher offers, namely, that of

informed consent, will be spoken of here as free informed consent.

One way of guarding against the misuse of the
person, then, is to grant him his right to free informed
consent (or dissent) with regard to that which is to
be done to him. Such a right is his by the fact of his
humanity. To deny him this right is to treat him as a
mere object or thing, a technique that is characteristic
of any type of misuse.

There are different circumstances that lie in the
way of free informed consent. Pressures within the
situation can jeopardize the patient's ability to offer
a free consent or dissent. These pressures may come
in the form of family pressures urging dissent rather
than consent, with the patient being fearful of going
against such pressure. The resulting consent or dissent is far from being free. Rather, it is pressured
and often the result of a fear of being rejected by the
pressuring element, which in itself can be a serious
matter, particularly in the case of the aged or crip-
pled who are virtually dependent upon the pressuring element. The wise physician will recognize such
pressures and will realize that in such a situation the
patient is incapable of free informed consent or dissent with regard to the experiment and thus is not a
fit subject for the experiment. Naturally, it is idealis-
tic to think or even to hope that any consent or dissent is given wholly free from pressures. Even when
external pressures from family and loved ones do
not exist, there may be pressure within the man him-

self wrought out of his own fear of what others would think were he to dissent. This is not to mention his own fear that he is not man enough to meet the request.

The attending physician must be aware of such pressures and know that a person under undue pressure, be it external or internal, is not a free person. He must know that such a person is highly subject to misuse, and he must be doubly cautious in deciding whether to use him as an experimental subject.

Obviously, free consent or dissent cannot be given by those who do not have the freedom of mind with which to decide. This necessarily includes the mentally defective, upon whom human experimentation is always subject to question.

Prerequisite to giving free informed consent, a man must understand the nature of the experiment and the part he will play as the experimental subject. Any explanation of the nature of the experiment should provide the patient with an understanding of the possible effects such an experiment will have on medical science in general and on him in particular. Medical science owes the experimental subject an intelligent and honest explanation regarding the use that is going to be made of his body and those organs and systems vital to his well-being. A common example of this is the responsibility of the medical scientist to give full explanation to the patient if, during the process of the experimentation, the patient will be under the influence of drugs or techniques that may alter his or her masculinity or femininity.

A burden is placed upon the doctor who seeks to obtain consent from his patient to use him as an experimental subject. The doctor needs to recognize this as a burden, for to recognize it as anything less is to take the issue of human experimentation too casually, as if it did not involve man in his suffering and pain. The doctor must bear the burden of determining whether he has been thoroughly honest with his patient and whether he has properly weighed the pressures confronting the patient in an effort to decide whether the patient is capable of giving free informed consent.

Just as certain situations exist that limit the patient's ability to give free consent or dissent, certain situations arise that prohibit the patient from giving informed consent. One's consent is informed to the extent that one has been informed about the nature of the experiment and the risks involved. Therefore, one situation which stands in the way of the patient's giving informed consent is that in which the doctor fails to give adequate information regarding the experiment and the risks, information necessary in order for a person to give such consent.

It is a generally accepted fact that minors and the mentally defective are unable to give informed consent. In the case of the minor, his age and his lack of maturity inhibit his ability to give such consent. The mentally defective person may be unable to cope with or to understand the information given him by the doctor, thus inhibiting him from giving informed consent. The giving of informed consent requires that one have the capacity to understand the risks involved in the experiment and the stability to cope with the situation. Again, the physician must be wise to those situations which involve a patient who is unable to understand the risks involved or to withstand emotionally the experiment. This patient, along with the patient who is under undue pressure, is highly susceptible to misuse. Such situations call for extreme caution and respect with regard to one's handling of the patient.

Dr. Beecher's second safeguard is important in assuring that the consent given is free informed consent. Without question, there are unwise investigators in the field of human experimentation. Witness the fact that some highly reputable research centers have been subject to criticism with regard to the unethical use of human subjects. "The celebrated Sloan-Kettering case where live cancer cells were injected into human subjects without their consent"[8] confirms the need for an intelligent, informed, conscientious, compassionate, responsible investigator in all experimentation involving human subjects. Such a safeguard is necessary to ensure that adequate and honest information has been given regarding the nature of the experiment and the risks involved, and to ascertain whether or not the person is sufficiently free of undue pressure to offer free consent and is intellectually and emotionally stable enough to give informed consent.

For the protection of the dignity and security of the individual, the patient must be granted his right to give free informed consent or dissent with regard to any experiment that is to be done to him. In granting man his right of free informed consent or dissent, medical science, in its use of man, treats man as an end in himself. Only as medical science treats man as an end in himself can human experimentation proceed without the patient fearing that he will become merely the object of medical science. Freedom from such fear is the right of any patient, and it is the moral duty of medical science to grant and protect this freedom.

Since the morality of human experimentation depends upon treating the patient as an end in himself, it is important to question what it means to treat one as an end in himself. There are two ways in particular of interpreting this. It may be interpreted to mean that the patient's physical well-being must be served from that which is to be done to him. This interprets the phrase narrowly, because there is the situation in which an experiment is done on a person as a result of his free consent, an experiment from which he knows that he cannot enjoy any physical benefit but for which he wishes to be used because of the valuable knowledge that can be gained for the benefit of others. There is something noble and gracious about such a person, who knows that because of his illness he cannot hope to benefit, but he can hope that the knowledge gained will give life to someone else. To say that such a person is not an end in himself is to deny the dimension of human life that is clothed in love and concern for the sufferings of others. To allow this person to be an experimental subject is to treat him as an end in himself, interpreting this more broadly to mean the right of a person to consent to an experiment from which he can physically benefit nothing but from which knowledge may be gained so that others need not suffer the same sickness and death.

This idea of treating man as an end in himself is more simply stated as treating man as a person. A person is not a mere object or thing, though one phase of man's relationship with medical science is that of his being the object through whom medical science gains much of its knowledge. In the words of Samuel Stumpf: "No one will suggest that there be no medical volunteers; the argument is simply that the moral conditions of the relationship be preserved wherein the subject is not merely used as a thing but treated as a person."[9]

THE EXPERIMENTAL NATURE OF ORGAN TRANSPLANTATION

Serious questioning has arisen in the mind of the general public and from various members of the medical profession owing to the rapid growth of organ transplantation surgery since the development of aza-thioprine (an immunosuppressive agent—an agent that helps to suppress the body's natural desire to reject foreign elements within its walls) in the early 1960's and particularly since the advent of cardiac transplantation surgery in December, 1967. In the face of such questioning and in the wake of the fear that man might become merely the object of scientific investigation, one must consider what constitutes the experimental nature of transplantation surgery and what is the purpose or goal of such surgery.

To begin with, organ transplantation surgery is experimental in that problems in surgical technique, postoperative patient care, and immunosuppressive therapy are still to be worked through. Of these, the *Journal of the American Medical Association* regards immunosuppressive therapy to be the major problem confronting transplantation surgery today. "Despite the advances made in immunosuppressive therapy, the problem of maintaining a viable organ in a hostile environment, without fatally compromising the host's ability to resist disease, remains the central problem of organ transplantation."[10]

The problem regarding immunosuppressive therapy may be summarized as follows: The body has a built-in mechanism or defense system whose function it is to fight off infection and any other foreign element that invades it. The physician knows that the defense system has been activated when he notes a rise in the patient's white cell count. Any person who has had a finger suppurate from the presence of a splinter has seen the body's defense system in action. The process of suppuration is the body's attempt to rid itself of the foreign element. Unfortunately, however, the body is unable to distinguish between the foreign element (such as the splinter or bacteria) that could destroy it and the foreign element (such as the transplanted heart) that is wont to restore life to it. Unable to distinguish between the foreign element that could destroy it and the one that could save it, the body reacts to the foreign organ implanted within its walls with the same furious desire to repel or reject it as it does to the presence of a splinter.

As a result of this defense system, the body will fight off or try to reject any foreign organ transplanted within its walls. This defense policy is spoken of medically as the immunological barrier and it exists between all human beings except identical twins. In order to continue transplanting organs, medical science had to develop drugs or some other method to suppress the host body's reaction of resisting the implanted organ. In the past fifteen years, various drugs have been developed that have proved instrumental in suppressing the immune reaction. These drugs are reasonably called immunosuppressive drugs, and they include azathioprine (Imuran), corticosteroids (prednisone in particular), and antilymphocyte serum (ALS) or antilymphocyte globulin (ALG).[11] The use of these immunosuppressive agents in renal (kidney) and cardiac (heart) transplantation surgery has made organ transplantations in man possible.

Immunosuppressive therapy, however, has a number of side effects. Among these is one that presently holds cardiac transplantation surgery to a research procedure. This side effect constitutes a "sharp reduction in the ability of the body to defend itself against bacterial, viral, and fungal invasion."[12] Just as the body is unable to distinguish between the foreign element that could destroy it and the foreign organ implanted within its walls to save it, it cannot, under the influence of immunosuppressive therapy, distinguish between being receptive to the implanted organ and being receptive to foreign elements, such as bacteria and viruses. This is the irony surrounding the body's defense system, an irony that must be broken if cardiac transplantation is to gain wide clinical acceptance. Dr. Helen Taussig, of the Johns Hopkins School of Medicine, writes regarding cardiac transplantation:

> Some day, we know not how soon or how late, we will know how a person can develop tolerance to one organ and still fight off other foreign substances and infections. Until such time, cardiac transplantation will remain a research procedure.[13]

In discussing the experimental nature of organ transplantation, we need to note that whereas cardiac transplantation surgery remains at the level of a research procedure and a clinical trial, renal transplantation surgery is rapidly gaining the status of a clinical procedure. Various reasons lie behind this distinction in status. The first successful renal transplantation surgery between human identical twins was performed in 1954.[14] This success was followed in 1959 by the first successful renal transplantation between other than identical twins (fraternal twins) as a result of "using total body irradiation in sub-

lethal dose to breach a moderate immunological barrier between this pair of fraternal twins." The current
state of renal transplantation (transplantation between unrelated donor and host) arose as a result of
the development of azathioprine, which is currently
used as a basic immunosuppressive agent in all organ
transplantations.[15] Valuable knowledge has been
gained since 1954 with regard to the tendency of the
body to reject the renal (kidney) graft and the use of
immunosuppressive therapy, to the extent that Dr.
Thomas Starzal at the Veterans Administration Hospital in Denver, Colorado, has recently achieved a
"95% one year survival rate in a group of unrelated
living donors."[16] Along with this figure it has been
estimated that since 1950, approximately 1,100 patients have survived out of the 2,100 who have
received renal grafts.[17]

The acceptance of renal transplantation surgery as
rapidly reaching the status of a clinical procedure
depends not alone on its success rate and the valuable
knowledge that has been gained regarding immunosuppressive therapy, but also upon two important
procedures that are at present peculiar to such surgery. In renal transplantation surgery, the rejection
reaction does not seem to be as furious as it is in
cardiac transplantation surgery. Further, when rejection appears inevitable, high doses of corticosteroids
may be used with relative success to reverse the rejection reaction.[18] The degree of rejection reversibility
that the renal graft enjoys does not seem to be the
case with cardiac grafts.

A second advantage (or peculiarity) that renal transplantation surgery enjoys over cardiac transplantation surgery is that of the removal of the transplant when total rejection appears inevitable. In abandoning the transplant, the renal graft is removed and the patient is maintained by dialysis (a process that involves circulating the patient's blood through an artificial kidney in order to "keep the electrolyte and water content of the body within constant limits and to eliminate certain waste products of protein metabolism"[19]) until another transplant can be carried out. As a result of the progress that has been made in the last twenty years regarding renal transplantation surgery, such surgery "is rapidly reaching the period when it can be considered a clinical procedure for the treatment of patients with renal disease."[20]

This is not the case with cardiac transplantation surgery. The cardiac transplantation surgeon, faced with a patient's inevitable rejection of the transplanted organ, does not have the option of abandoning the cardiac graft to the use of a machine comparable in cardiac care to the artificial kidney in renal care. In the event that severe organ rejection is inevitable, the surgeon is left to decide whether or not to let the patient succumb to the destruction of the organ through rejection or to administer large doses of potentially lethal immunosuppressive drugs and in so doing possibly destroy entirely the body's ability to war against such foreign elements as bacteria and viruses.

Since the status of cardiac transplantation surgery

is that of a research procedure, one is right to question whether the widespread use of such an experimental method is justified. Such questioning has arisen within the ranks of the medical profession itself, one critic stating that "as long as rejection remains a principal problem, it should be researched in dogs and small animals until there is reasonable assurance that the major difficulties have been solved."[21]

In trying to decide whether or not the widespread use of such an experimental method is justified, one must weigh a number of things in the balance. To begin with, one must ask, What is the goal or purpose of such a procedure? One would hope and expect that both the lay public and the medical profession would recoil from the widespread use of such a drastic procedure if it were merely for the acquisition of knowledge.

Though valuable knowledge has been gained through recent cardiac transplantation surgical attempts, the mere acquisition of knowledge is not the goal of this surgical technique. Rather, "the goal of cardiac transplantation is long-term restoration of a critically ill patient to a productive and personally enjoyable life."[22] It is hard to say that this goal has ever been reached owing to the relative newness of cardiac transplantation surgery, though some patients have been restored to a satisfactory life for over a year.

One might question how such a goal is ever to be reached except through the continuation of cardiac transplantations. Such a question is warranted, and it is a fact that a goal cannot be reached unless one makes a serious attempt to reach it. But it is also true that a man at times sets out prematurely to achieve his goal. This is to say that there are times when a man sets out to achieve his goal before he has taken time to master sufficiently the procedural technique or to gain the knowledge necessary to make the achievement of that goal a viable possibility. This question of prematurity is one that must be weighed in the balance in deciding whether or not the widespread use of such an experimental method is justified. In testing a new jet, the test pilot gains knowledge as to whether and to what extent that jet should be adopted for practical use. The pilot is careful to respect the knowledge he gains, realizing that his judgment, or lack of judgment, affects the protection or destruction of human life. In the same manner, the knowledge that the surgeon gains in performing the cardiac transplantations and in observing his patient during his period of postoperative care and possible organ rejection should tell him whether and to what extent the procedure may be adopted for practical use.

One piece of knowledge that medical science is aware of and must deal with is the deleterious side effects of one immunosuppressive drug in particular. Immunosuppressive therapy, which is implemented in an attempt to enable the body to tolerate a foreign organ, has shown itself, in some cases, to be intolerant of man as a whole person. In addition to reducing the body's ability to fight off infection, this particular immunosuppressive agent has shown itself to be destructive of man's psychological well-being. This poses a particular problem in cardiac transplantation surgery where the patient is likely to be subject to immunosuppressive therapy for the remainder of his life. The question of what a new heart may do to the mind has serious medical and moral import. One must seriously question the type of reasoning that lies behind the attempt to heal a man physically when his mind stands to be sacrificed in the process. Dr. Donald T. Lunde, of Stanford University in California, has reported that three of nine patients who underwent cardiac transplantation surgery at Stanford in 1968 developed postoperative psychosis.[23] One forty-five-year-old man, after receiving a heart from a twenty-year-old donor, announced to his friends the celebration of his twentieth birthday. Another recipient announced an intention to live up to the "sterling reputation" of his good-citizen donor. In the third case the male recipient of a woman's heart expressed great fear of feminization, though his fear was somewhat lessened upon learning that women live longer than men.[24] Lunde, a psychiatrist and consultant to surgeon Norman Shumway's transplant team, reports these three cases as representing some of the less severe psychological changes that have been observed. In a series of thirteen transplants over a sixteen-month period "three of the nonsurvivors became psychotic before they died last year. And two others have become psychotic this year."[25] It should be noted that all the transplant patients mentioned here had been subjected to careful screening for the detection of any mental abnormalities before having been accepted as potential transplant recipients.

The question that must be asked, and already has been asked by some members of the medical profession, is whether or not medical science is justified in using a drug that in healing a man physically can destroy him mentally.

It seems ironic to call a cardiac transplantation a success when the surgery and the postoperative therapy render the patient psychotic. The same lack of reasoning seen here is also seen in the report that says the surgery was a success because the organ was functioning properly at the time of the patient's death; death itself was due to a viral infection that the body was helpless against owing to the immunosuppressive therapy and its effect on the body's defense system. Medical science must come to see itself as being in an age in which it must judge success by the quality of life it gives a patient and not merely by the fact that it prolongs the patient's life.

There is little quality to life when a man has no control over his mood or cognition. To build up a man physically and tear him down mentally, or to restore him to physical well-being and destroy his psychological well-being, is a monstrous deed for which any doctor performing it must hold himself personally accountable.

Whether such knowledge as this tells the surgeon that the procedure should be discontinued in humans, or whether it tells him that it should be continued in humans but limited to those fatally ill patients for whom there is no other method of treatment, is largely up to his discretion. In interpreting this knowledge, however, it is the physician's moral responsibility to interpret it for the promotion of the well-being of his patients.

Here again, the promotion of human well-being is seen to be both medicine's purpose and its dilemma, in that there is no criterion whereby the physician knows what the promotion of human well-being means or requires in each situation. When the knowledge that the surgeon gains shows the risk to human life and limb to be high, he may interpret the knowledge as telling him that it is time he return to experimentation on animals alone. In another case, however, though the risk is high, he may interpret the knowledge as a signal to go ahead because of the possibility, however remote, that the operation could save a patient who has only this chance and this moment left.

It is difficult to try to justify the widespread use of any new procedure that is drastic in its nature and can be equally drastic in its outcome. Perhaps one approaches medical science improperly in asking it to justify itself. Perhaps one should look to each individual situation and ask whether medical science has the right to deny the dying patient the only hope for life he has left. On the other hand, lack of wisdom in knowing when not to go forward can destroy the hope of the many through continual failure.

Caution need not be a barrier in the way of progress. Indeed, caution itself may be the way forward. One physician who is intimately concerned lest the prematurity of the widespread use of cardiac transplantation surgery exact a disproportionate loss in human well-being has said: "I hope that physicians and surgeons will proceed with extreme caution until such time as a cardiac transplant will not announce the imminence of death, but will offer the patient the probability of a return to a useful life for a number of years."[26]

There have been times and there will be times when the acquisition of knowledge will be costly to human life and limb. This is a fact of human existence and progress, but the acquisition of knowledge need not be and must not be dehumanizing. There is a difference between the medical procedure that may be costly to human life and limb and that procedure which is dehumanizing. An example of the prior procedure includes the man who offers himself as an experimental subject, knowing that physically he can gain nothing for himself, but may, through the knowledge gained, offer much to others. This is far different from the procedure that is dehumanizing, an example of which is the situation in which a man is not permitted to decide when and to what extent he will be used as the object of scientific investigation. Such a procedure is dehumanizing in that it does not grant or recognize man's right to give free informed consent or dissent to that experiment of which he is to be a part.

Medicine's Quest
to Redefine Death

AN IRONY OF MEDICAL ADVANCE

There was a time in the history of the practice of medicine when the question of what constitutes death did not pose the perplexing problem that it does today. The doctor, armed with but a few medicines and with a limited amount of scientific knowledge, had at his disposal relatively few lifesaving methods or techniques. In his mind he carried the knowledge he had gained from what medical texts and medical education were available to him. In his black bag he carried syringes and needles, a few vials of medicine, tongue depressors, pills and medications, and a few crude surgical instruments. He was neither the guarantor of a long life nor of an easy death. But for all that he lacked and for all the limitations that his time in history placed upon him, no doubt he came closer to understanding the meaning of life and death than has any doctor in the years after him.

The so-called heroic extraordinary methods of prolonging life, which are at home in hospitals of this age, were not a part of his bag. His age was truly the age of medicine, and when the medicine failed, the patient died—except for those instances of a sudden change for the better explainable only in terms of a miracle. This is not to say that the process of dying was an easy one, devoid of pain and suffering. This was not the case. Pain and suffering are often closely affiliated with death, and perhaps they were even more so at that time when pain-relieving and pain-suppressing drugs were not available than they are now when such drugs are in daily use. The doctor's practice, like the age in which he lived, was simplistic. He used, as best he could, the meager tools and knowledge that he had in an effort to promote human well-being, and when the odds of disease and suffering outweighed what he was capable of doing, he waited. In the end, when the odds had taken their toll, he was able to say, "The patient is dead."

The days of the country doctor and his black bag are virtually a thing of the past. Gone also is the simplistic nature of his practice and his age. In its place stand the scientific knowledge and technological genius that are a hallmark of the practice of medicine today. Such knowledge and genius have benefited both the practitioner and the patient and yet they have also complicated the doctor's task of determining when a patient is dead. For all that has been gained, medical science has sacrificed whatever certainty it had in the past regarding the proclamation of the event of death. The stark face of death that stared coldly into the eyes of the bygone country

doctor wears many masks today. The resuscitator and
cardiac pacemaker can mask death until the doctor is
confused as to whether he is dealing with a living
patient or with an unburied corpse. The irony that has
come as a result of recent medical advances is well
expressed in an editorial entitled "What and When
Is Death?":

> When all is said and done, it seems ironic that
> the end point of existence, which ought to be
> as clear and sharp as in a chemical titration,
> should so defy the power of words to describe
> it and the power of men to say with certainty,
> "It is here."[27]

THE PROCESS OF DYING

Medical scientists—physicians and researchers—
are involved in the task of redefining death and establishing a set of criteria by which death is to be determined. In a paper entitled "What Is Death?" Frank J.
Ayd describes the sequence of death or the process
of dying. Such a paper stands as an informative pro-
logue to medicine's quest to redefine death.

Ayd refers to the sequence of death as "an orderly
progression from clinical death to brain death, to
biological death, to cellular death."[28]

Clinical death, as the first stage in this progression,
occurs "when the body's vital functions—respiration
and heartbeat—wane and finally cease."[29] Depending
upon the cause of the clinical death, this first step in
the sequence may be reversed through resuscitative

measures and the patient restored to an active and meaningful life. An example of a reversal of clinical death and the restoration of a person may be seen in the case of the child who has drowned and is pulled out of the water limp and apparently lifeless, without heartbeat and respiration. The cessation of heartbeat and respiration denote clinical death. The child, however, is restored by the action of a well-trained lifeguard who immediately and successfully initiates mouth-to-mouth resuscitation and cardiac massage. Heartbeat and respiration are restored, and the child's life is saved.

Such a reversal of clinical death is not, however, always possible. For example, the heart and lungs may be injured to the extent that resuscitative measures are in vain. The child who in climbing a tree slips and falls to the ground, sustaining massive puncture wounds of the heart and lungs in the fall, may suffer injuries to the extent that cardiac and respiratory functioning cannot be revitalized. In the wake of clinical death (the cessation of heartbeat and respiration), the child incurs brain death in that the brain suffocates owing to a lack of oxygenation. As a result of brain death the child suffers biological death, which is denoted by the loss of organ function. The child passes through the entire sequence of death, and his life is extinct.

In the third type of case, clinical death may be reversed but with permanent brain damage having occurred. Such cases present a moral dilemma for medical science. Time is of the essence in initiating resuscitative measures on one who has suffered clinical death if partial or total brain functioning is not to be lost. After cardiac and respiratory arrest (clinical death), brain death follows quickly. Under normal temperature conditions, the human brain cannot survive loss of oxygen for more than ten minutes.[30] This is not to say that clinical death cannot be reversed after a ten-minute lapse. Rather, it is to say that clinical death may not be reversed after such a time lapse without brain damage and possible brain death resulting. An example of this is the case of a thirteen-year-old boy who had been trapped in a cave-in. The boy was without oxygen for about thirty minutes before his rescue. After being taken to a hospital, the boy underwent resuscitative therapy, and his heartbeat was restored. Clinical death had been reversed, but severe, permanent brain damage resulted from anoxia.[31] Because of the severity of the brain damage, the boy's respiration was dependent upon artificial means, and because of the permanent nature of the damage, he would be unable to breathe of his own accord again. This case exemplifies a situation in which resuscitory measures were started after the critical time lapse, with clinical life being restored but with permanent brain damage having occurred.

From these examples it can be seen that clinical death need not necessarily mean the death of the person, though it can lead to his death. The boy who drowned was restored to life, whereas the boy who sustained massive injuries to the chest died as a result of those injuries. On the other hand, the reversal of clinical death does not always mean the restoration of the patient to a level of life that one would want to call human life.

With regard to clinical death, it is generally the practice of physicians today to try to reverse clinical death through resuscitative means. In fact, it is quite natural that one tries to resuscitate another who has stopped breathing. Take, for example, the mother who applies mouth-to-mouth resuscitation to her infant or the workman who tries to resuscitate his friend who has touched a high-voltage cable. The passion to save the life of one who has stopped breathing is a quite common passion and fortunately so. The moral dilemma that the doctor faces does not surround the decision to resuscitate one who has stopped breathing. Rather, it involves the decision of postponing clinical death through artificial means when irreversible brain death has occurred. This is to say that the moral dilemma involves the decision to continue the use of artificial sustainers when the patient's brain is dead.

In an age in which artificial sustainers may be used to sustain almost without limit a person whose brain is dead, a pressing need has arisen to understand the place of the brain in human life and the meaning and importance of brain death.

Traditionally the heart has been recognized as the seat of life and love. To witness this, one need only explore some of the poetry of the past. Today it is time to sing of the brain the praises that have been sung of the heart.

It is said that one suffers a broken heart through the rebuke given by a loved one. The meaning of this cannot be, in the literal sense, that one's heart has been broken or torn apart but that one knows with his or her mind that he or she has disturbed or let the loved one down. It is not the heart that carries the burden of such rebuke but the mind. This is analogous to the situation of the mother who has lost a son in war. It is not her heart (a muscle that pumps blood through the body) that knows of such a loss but her mind. The mind knows, and if the heart grows faint, it is not through any knowledge it has of the loss, but through a command from the brain. It is not the heart that knows the joy of love but the mind. The heart, an obedient servant to the mind, may jump for the joy of the love the mind knows, but it cannot offer its own show of love in response. The heart is but a muscle and a pump, one organ among many. Human life and human love, like hope and the future, belong to the conscious world of man or to man's world of knowing. The implication here is that human life has not alone to do with the beat of the heart but with the knowledge that one is alive. It is by his brain that a man walks, laughs, talks, and cries. If one thinks this foolish, ponder for a moment the situation of the child or adult with a damaged or disturbed mind. Witness the moron, idiot, or imbecile, and ask what deficiency or disease of the heart muscle is the cause of such a manner of life.

The romanticized conception of the heart as the seat of life and love is being challenged today. No doubt it will take years before the mystique of the heart is to be seen for what it is. Medically, the heart is but tissue and nerves working together as a pump. Such a pumping device is vital to life, but the action alone of its pumping does not make the life that it sustains human life. This pump may be kept functioning by artificial means long after the patient has lost all sensibility and voluntary or involuntary movement. Because of this, one needs to realize that though the heart (or a pumping device like it) is vital to life, human life amounts to more than heartbeat and respiration.

Brain function is integral to the authentically human level of life. Man's possession of a brain sets him apart from vegetable life, and his capacity to reason with his brain sets him apart from animal life. Human life, seen in this way, depends upon a brain that endows man with the capacity to reason. When such a capacity is destroyed owing to the destruction of a portion of the brain or to total brain death, one begins to question seriously whether or not such a person is alive in a fully human sense.

This idea of the importance of brain function as a criterion of human life has led some within the medical profession to uphold the position that when man's brain is dead human life is gone. For this reason the question of what constitutes brain death has a serious import in medicine's quest to redefine death.

It has already been seen that brain death is the second stage in the sequence of death and it occurs in the wake of clinical death unless resuscitative measures are initiated immediately. The brain undergoes its own process of dying. In the words of Ayd, "The brain also dies in progressive steps."[32] As a victim of anoxia (oxygen starvation), the brain dies by component parts, starting with the cortex, moving to the midbrain (diencephalon), and ending with the brainstem.[33] Brain death then, in simpler terms, means the death of each of the component parts of the brain. "Ultimately, when all the components of the brain are dead, biological death, or permanent extinction of bodily life, occurs."[34]

The painful and often cruel fact about the functioning of the brain is that through an injury or illness part of the brain may be permanently destroyed (cases of partial brain death), while the other component parts continue functioning. This is because the brain is composed of higher and lower levels. The higher levels have to do with man's consciousness; the lower levels with nervous system and cardiorespiratory or heart-lung functioning. As the result of an injury, the patient may suffer cortical death or death of the cortex (controlling the higher level of brain functioning), while lower-level functioning continues. Through the loss of higher-level functioning, the patient sustains permanent loss of consciousness. Medically and legally, however, he is not dead. In such a case, cardiorespiratory function may continue of its own accord, or it may need the aid of artificial sustainers. One test used to determine whether there is any respiratory function when there is doubt is to remove the artificial sustainer to see if the patient attempts to breathe of his own accord. The word "attempts" is important here. The test is not to see whether or not the patient can breathe of his own accord. It is to see if the patient makes an effort to breathe of his own accord, regardless of whether he succeeds or fails. Any attempt to breathe on the part of the patient, though he fails, is taken to be a sign of life, and doctors generally see themselves morally obligated to return the patient to the use of the sustainer.

Examples of this type of existence frequent the medical journals and are exemplified by the case of a twenty-one-year-old Montreal woman, Lise Dagenais, who died recently after being in a coma for twelve years as the result of injuries sustained in an auto accident.[35] Though this woman had no sensibility for this entire period, medically and legally, though dying, she was not dead.

The purpose in mentioning this type of case is not that of establishing ethical guidelines as to what should or should not be done in such situations, but rather to show that a person may be the victim of irreversible brain damage without being the victim of brain death. Irreversible brain death is a very restrictive category that entails the irreversible destruction of each component part of the brain.

As a result of brain death, bodily life ceases. A dead brain is powerless to sustain bodily life. As bodily life dies, cellular death takes place. Because the various organs and elements of the body are of different cellular compositions, some of them will die more rapidly than others. This extended period of cellular death is witnessed by the growth of the fingernails and hair for a period of time after the death of the person.

The process of dying involves the sequence of various kinds of death from clinical death to cellular death. The patient may have begun the process of dying and yet he may still be saved. The onset of the process of dying does not necessarily mean that the process will be completed, resulting in the extinction of life.[36]

THREE APPROACHES TO A REDEFINITION

The task of redefining death is no easy one. At best it is a burden, and in the opinion of some it is a burden that medical science is incapable of handling. To the task of redefining death has been brought the question of whether or not a science can define something whose meaning it does not know. Medical scientists do not know the full meaning of life and death— neither does the pastor, the philosopher, nor the lawyer, for that matter. At most, the medical scientist can isolate and attempt to interpret to the pastor, philosopher, and lawyer certain life signs which denote that an object has the characteristics of being alive. In like manner, they can distinguish a sequence of events, the termination of which makes life extinct. But beyond being able to recognize certain life signs and certain death signs, the scientist must grant the meaning of life and death to be a mystery.

Medical scientists can reproduce or initiate human life in a test tube by bringing together sperm and ovum. They witness the mystery of life, however, in that they are unable to go behind the sperm and the ovum to produce human life. The fate of science is that it must start with something in order to produce something in return. It cannot start with nothing and hope to produce anything. Where life comes from is part of the mystery in which medical science is involved but of which it is not the master. If medical men know God or if they have ever felt themselves to be in the presence of a power that surpasses their scientific scrutiny, it is no doubt at those times when they witness the beginning of life or of life's end.

The task of medical scientists in redefining death, though a burden and though difficult, is within the realm of human possibilities. The fact that they do not know the meaning of life and death simply means that the redefinition they arrive at will not have come from any knowledge of the meaning of life and death. Rather, any such definition will be born out of their knowledge of the physiological signs whose presence denotes life and whose absence denotes death. These signs will be the material of any redefinition determined and approved by medical science. Since medical science can deal only with empirical facts, the definition that results will be one weighted with measurable data.

In an attempt to redefine death and to establish a set of criteria by which death may be determined, three schools of thought have arisen. Paul Ramsey distinguishes these three schools. The first would interpret death to be brain death and would use the electroencephalograph exclusively, or almost exclusively, in determining death. The second school also holds the meaning of death to be brain death but uses a number of other tests in addition to the electroencephalogram in determining a state of irreversible brain death. The third school urges that the tests for determining death be improved, but it sees death in the traditional terms of permanent cessation of heart, lung, and brain activity.[37]

The first of the positions, which Paul Ramsey characterizes as the most radical, is the only one to rely upon the criterion of brain function alone in the determination of death. Perhaps the most perplexing question about this position is that of the constitution of the criteria of death outside of an isoelectric reading on the electroencephalograph. Such a position can easily leave one with an uncertainty as to what is meant by brain death.

The second position, on the other hand, spells out what constitutes brain death by the methods it uses to determine such death. This position is offered by the Ad Hoc Committee of the Harvard Medical School. The report of this committee comes under the title of "A Definition of Irreversible Coma."[38] The committee's use of the term "irreversible coma" is important and needs to be examined. Such a phrase can be confusing in that an irreversible coma has at times meant that a patient had suffered the permanent destruction of that part of the brain (the brain's higher level of functioning) which controlled his consciousness. Through the destruction of that portion of the brain the patient would lapse into unconsciousness, though other vital functions such as nervous system and cardiorespiratory functioning would perhaps continue. The patient's state would be that of being in a coma, and an irreversible coma at that if the destruction of the higher level of brain functioning was of a permanent nature. This is, however, precisely what the Harvard Committee does *not* mean by irreversible coma or brain death. An irreversible coma means the permanent loss of both the higher and the lower levels of brain functioning, thus entailing a permanent state of unconsciousness and the permanent and total loss of cardiorespiratory functioning.

The Harvard Committee, under the chairmanship of Dr. Henry K. Beecher, has set down four criteria whose presence characterizes a permanently nonfunctioning brain. They are: unreceptivity and unresponsitivity, no movements or breathing, no reflexes, a flat electroencephalogram.[39] A patient with an irreversible coma (brain death) will be totally unresponsive to external stimuli and inner need. Intensely painful stimuli, which would normally cause a person to yell, pull away, or increase his rate of breathing, will elicit no response from the patient. He will have fixed, dilated pupils. All eye movement,

including blinking, will be absent. The total absence
of these movements may be tested by turning the
patient's head and by irrigating his ears with ice
water. He will neither notice nor respond to plantar
stimulation, such as tickling the sole of the foot or
pricking it with a pin. Harmful stimulation will evoke
no reflexes. In watching the patient, one will notice
that he no longer swallows, yawns, or vocalizes.
Neither eye nor throat reflexes can be established.
He will not breathe or move. Close observation of the
patient by physicians and the patient's inability to
breathe of his own accord within a three-minute
period after the respirator is turned off establish his
inability to breathe spontaneously. The patient's flat
electroencephalogram will further confirm his state
of irreversible coma. Brain death, however, may be
declared without the use of the electroencephalogram. In the view of the Harvard Committee, the
patient's unreceptivity and unresponsitivity, loss of
reflexes, cessation of breathing and movement, and,
when available, flat electroencephalogram are indica-
tive of brain death. The committee suggests that all
tests for determining irreversible coma are to be repeated at least twenty-four hours later with no
change, and that the patient's temperature is not to
be under 90°F. (32.2°C.), nor is he to be under the
influence of central nervous system depressants. If
these conditions exist, the tests cannot be held to be
conclusive of the patient's death.[40]

It is important to note that this position lists the
electroencephalogram last and grants it the value of

being confirmatory. Unlike the first position, it does not hold the electroencephalograph reading to be the determinant of brain death. The procedure for determining brain death may be carried out in the absence of electroencephalographic monitoring. When such monitoring is not available, the absence of cerebral functioning may be determined by purely clinical signs that the committee has outlined or by the "absence of circulation as judged by standstill of blood in the retinal vessels, or by absence of cardiac activity."[41] When electroencephalographic monitoring is available, the test serves to confirm the information gained by the other tests.

Such a method of determining brain death or irreversible coma substantiates the fact that medical science knows what death is only in terms of the measurable. The patient's ability to be receptive and responsive, his ability to move and to breathe, and his ability to reflex is tested, and then his measured failure or measured success denotes either a state of being dead or of being alive.

A word may be said with regard to this method of determining brain death as being safe. Its safety is to be seen in that there is no need for guesswork or room for an assumption regarding death. The patient is not assumed or guessed to be dead. He is seen to be dead. The committee's criteria for determining brain death take away the shady edges and get the doctor off the limb, so to speak. A method such as this may be seen to be essential to medical science in that a science can only know the fact of something by the measure of it. Death, as such, is a demonstrable fact.

The criteria set forth by the Harvard Committee not only serve medical science in the act of determining the event of death but they also set the limits of what condition in man denotes death. The establishment of these criteria provides a redefinition of death.

In regard to the proclamation of the event of death, the committee urges that the respirator be turned off only *after* death is declared by the physician-in-charge along with one or more other physicians who have had a direct involvement in the case.[42] This procedure acts as a necessary precautionary measure against certain accusations that could arise. It is a precaution against the accusation that the patient died as a result of the respirator having been turned off. It is also a precaution against the accusation that the doctor-in-charge had an ulterior motive in declaring his patient dead. This in particular is a precaution against the accusation, which could easily arise today, to the effect that the doctor declared the patient dead because of the urgent need for a donor heart. The need for such a precautionary measure is already evident and will undoubtedly become more pronounced as organ transplantation surgery continues.

The third position for redefining death is in keeping with the traditional concept or meaning of death. This position does not shift to a position calling for death to be redefined through a definition of brain death, but it holds to a reasonable tension among brain, heart, and lung functioning. Its purpose is not that of the Harvard Committee of redefining death in terms of brain death or irreversible coma. It does, however, share with the committee an intent to clarify and enumerate the various tests used to determine death. Dr. Vincent J. Collins stresses the importance of brain, heart, and lung functioning as integrated rather than as independent functions.

> It is the whole organism, representing the sum of the structural parts, all integrated functionally, which establish the existence of life. To these are added a supreme integrative action by the central nervous system. Thus, by the total integrative process, there emerges a being greater than the parts called man.[43]

The integrated functioning of the structural parts and the central nervous system is here stressed over and against any independent functioning of any one or two parts. For Collins the integrated failure of the structural parts and central nervous system is integral to death just as their integrated functioning is integral to life. Death, in this manner of understanding it, is not a matter of the failure of one or two organs. Death, rather, is a process involving the integrated failure of the bodily parts and systems. As such, the cessation of heartbeat and respiration does not necessarily denote the death of the person. For Dr. Collins the first stage in the process of dying involves a "functional disorder or disequilibration"[44] comparable to

Ayd's first progression in the sequence of death: that of clinical death.

In an attempt to determine what denotes the death of a person, Collins proposes a "dying score." He bases this dying score on five physiologic functions: cerebral, reflex, respiratory, circulatory, and cardiac, with death meaning "the cessation of these integrated and (in that order) dependent functions."[45] Each of these five functions is given its own score. For example, if cerebral functioning is present, it is given the score of "two." If it is potential rather than present, it is given the score of "one." If, on the other hand, cerebral functioning is absent, it is given the score of "zero." Each of the five physiologic functions is scored in this manner. Death is taken to be conclusive when each function shows a zero score. When the total score is five or more, there is life potential in the patient. This score, it needs to be noted, says nothing about the quality of the life potential; it merely admits that life is potential and the person is alive. A score of under five, on the other hand, represents " 'impending' or 'presumptive' death."[46]

Perhaps the most obvious similarity among these three attempts at redefining death is the precision with which they seek to determine the event of death. The third attempt is one of calculated precision. The first seeks the definiteness of a graph. The Harvard Committee seeks to establish certain criteria as the measures by which death is to be held conclusive. Such precision and definiteness may in the future free medical science from certain problems and accusations with which it has been confronted in the past few years. With regard to organ transplantation and the proclamation of death, two of these positions would require that the heart of the donor had stopped beating before death could be declared and the organ removed. The importance of such a requirement is already being felt and will be felt to a greater extent as heart transplantations become more numerous. Such precision and definiteness, however, do not solve all the problems that medical science faces with regard to what constitutes the death of a person and the proclamation of the event of death.

REDEFINING DEATH: THE MORAL ISSUE

The quest of medical scientists to redefine death is the result of an irony of medical advance. For all that medicine has gained in scientific and technological knowledge, it has sacrificed whatever certainty it had with regard to the proclamation of the event of death. Medicine's ability to prolong life by artificial means has complicated its task of defining death. This dilemma of medical advance is further complicated by the dawn of cardiac transplantation surgery.

In cardiac transplantation surgery (as in transplantation surgery involving any unpaired vital organ— for example, the heart as contrasted with the kidneys) the life of one person depends upon the death of another. The question of a redefinition of death and the establishment of certain criteria by which death is to be determined cannot be avoided if the transplantation of unpaired vital organs is to continue.

The question of the redefinition of death is strictly medical in one sense and moral in another. It is a medical question in that only medical science itself can redefine death for its own technical purposes. It is not the task of philosophy, theology, or law, no matter how passionately concerned they are about the necessity for redefinition. It is a question that medical scientists must deal with and recognize as a question involving moral issues. It is a moral question in that it involves the issue of respect for the human being. The need to obtain unpaired vital organs is great. Greater still, however, is the need to respect the rights of the dying person. To redefine death so that the doctor will know with certainty when death has occurred and thus when it would be permissible for him to remove unpaired organs is one thing. To redefine death for the purpose of obtaining more organs for transplantation is quite another thing.

The reason and intention behind the attempt to redefine death are moral issues. To redefine death and to establish a set of criteria by which death may be determined in an attempt to understand better what constitutes that condition called "death" and when it occurs is morally justified in this age of artificial sustainers in which certain life signs may be prolonged indefinitely. To redefine death with the intent of storing up viable organs for transplantation is again another question.

Medicine, in its attempt to redefine death, must search itself to the depths lest the proclamation of the event of death become merely a tool in the hands of the doctor. Man is to be declared dead because he is no longer alive. The need for a transplant organ may be coincidental with another's death, but the need for a transplant organ must never be the reason for the proclamation of another man's death.

In an age in which the life of one depends upon the death of another, life itself must be held in waiting. No doubt this will come as a bitter dose to a science that seeks to save lives. The transgression of this principle, however, could be more bitter still. It could be the cup of hemlock of medical science. How man, in his sickness and in his health, looks upon medical science depends, in part, upon how medical science looks upon man's death.

The moral issues surrounding the redefinition of death amount to more than the reason and intention behind any attempted redefinition. The redefinition that medical science arrives at is in itself a moral issue. This is exemplified by the fact that the redefinition of death plays a part in shaping the concept of man that medical science holds. It is precisely because of this fact that any redefinition of death is itself a moral issue. The concept that a person has of man determines to a large extent how that person will treat man. In like manner, the concept that medical scientists have of man will bear directly on how they deal with and handle man in his sickness and his need. The concept of man is of crucial significance to the conduct of medical scientists in dealing with those who seek their help.

If man's life and death are explained only in terms of those physiological life signs whose presence denotes life and whose absence denotes death, the temptation arises to see man merely as a collect of those physiological life signs. The importance of such a concept of man and its implication cannot be overlooked. It is, in fact, just such a concept as this (as a collect of certain physiological life signs) that has given rise to what are sadly but logically called "vegetable wards." Such a concept of man urges the artificial prolongation of those physiological life signs. Whether doctors see themselves morally obligated and morally justified in prolonging by artificial means the life of a hopelessly ill patient depends upon their concept of man. Herein lies the moral issue. The medical care and treatment of man are fashioned out of the concept of man on the part of medical scientists.

The concept of man that holds him to be a collect of physiological life signs is a concept of natural science. It is based upon measurable and easily recognizable factors. It is only natural that medical science would bear and nurture such a concept. And yet, a concept of man that propagates the artificial prolongation of a few life signs for an indefinite period when all hope and future are already dead is morally questionable. Does not a concept that prohibits man's right to die with dignity fall short of being morally justified? Is it not, perhaps, the moral duty of medical scientists to seek a redefinition of death that would recognize and guarantee man's right to die with dignity?

A concept of man that holds him to be uniquely different from all other forms of life, rather than a mere collect of physiological life signs, has much to offer medical science in this day of medical genius and technological skill. It is precisely the question of what constitutes the human dimension of life that torments the mind of anyone who has ever seen a loved one who, in his or her illness, has passed into a vegetative state.

The human dimension of life has naturally to do with those aspects of human life which distinguish it from all other forms of life. Perhaps the most obvious aspect is that of man's capacity for reason and rationality. Neither animal life nor vegetable life shares this capacity. Man's gift of such a capacity separates him from all other forms of life. It constitutes that dimension of a man's life referred to as the authentically and peculiarly human dimension of life.

A fact that is crucial with regard to the human dimension of life and with regard to man in his illness and injury is the fact that through a serious illness or injury this dimension of life may be destroyed (this is to say, prior to brain death). In such a case, the human dimension of life is extinguished (constituting the destruction of man's capacity for reason and rationality) though a few physiological life signs may still be manifested, depending upon the state of the brain and the amount of brain destruction. It is true that the presence of a physiological life sign (for example, respiration) denotes life. But does the mere presence of a physiological life sign necessarily denote the presence of human life? Of course it does not. The mere fact that a body with a human form respires of its own accord or through the aid of an artificial sustainer is not enough to establish the presence of or existence of human life. "Vegetable wards" are populated with such forms, forms that are devoid of the human dimension of life as a result of severe injury or illness. The human forms in those wards partake of a vegetable level of life—a level that is inactive, passive, and unthinking. In resuscitating such a body, the biological activities of the organs are sustained, but human life is neither retained nor regained. Life may persist in the absence of the human dimension of life. Human life, however, can be neither retained nor regained once the human dimension of life has been destroyed. Patients in such a condition deserve loving care and consideration. But is it not proper, or is it too much to ask of a science, that man should be permitted to die when the dimension of his life that gave him the distinction of having been human has passed away? When this dimension of life has been destroyed, there is, humanly speaking, neither quality of life nor potential life quality. There is mere physiological existence devoid of hope and future. Man, in such a state of existence, deserves to be kept clean and warm. But does he not also deserve to pass beyond such a state of existence through being permitted to die?

Death, which medical science so often sees as its personal defeat, is but life's natural end. Man's birth ordains his death—as a man is born, so shall he die. Death, medicine's defeat, is man's right. And who can deny that it is a most blessed right when he has seen another in a state of existence devoid of human dimension, meaning, quality, or hope?

A life devoid of its human dimension is but a ghost of what once was. Not until medical science realizes that human life exists only in the presence of the human dimension of life will it be able to give up this ghost. Only as doctors see man to be more than a collect of physiological life signs will they respect the fact that the human being may be dead though the body lives on. Medical science has too long played with the ghost, giving to it its time and energy and technological genius. Time and energy spent have a lesson to teach, but only if the spender is a wise student. Physicians must seek the wisdom to know what man is and how human life differs from all other forms of life. Any wisdom short of this sees human life as something less than God made it.

Whether physicians see themselves morally obligated to prolong life by artificial means depends upon their concept of man. If their concept is that he is merely a collect of physiological life signs, they will easily see themselves obligated to sustain life artificially up to and including the last physiological life sign. If, on the other hand, the medical concept of man is one based upon an understanding of the human dimension of life and the dependence of the existence of human life on that dimension, physicians may well see themselves morally justified and even morally obligated to permit death by disavowing the use of artificial sustainers once the human dimension of life has been destroyed.

How physicians deal with and treat man depends upon their concept of man. Their concept of man and their understanding of what constitutes death are each dependent upon the other. Medicine's attempt to redefine death is shaped by, and in turn shapes, its concept of man. Upon medicine's redefinition of death and its concept of man depends how physicians will treat man in the future. Medicine's quest to redefine death must not be taken too lightly. Man's well-being depends upon the outcome of this quest.

The Gift of Life
(Organ Procurement: Recipient Selection)

DAWN OF A NEW DAY AND ITS LIMITATIONS

The history of medicine reads of a practice that has been confronted with an unlimited number of limitations. The history of the practice of medicine, however, reads beyond the limitations. It goes on to read of how a practice has surpassed its momentary limitations by means of its own knowledge and genius. A few examples are illustrative of this. Think how limited medical science once was in controlling bacterial infection. Then came penicillin. Think, again, of how limited medical science was in exploring the body's skeletal system. Then the X-ray was developed. Poliomyelitis was a dread disease of the late 1940's and early 1950's. Jonas Salk developed a vaccine, and for today's school children polio is but a page in a history book.

Today medical science is confronted with numerous limitations peculiar to this moment of scientific and technological advance. It has only limited knowledge of the body's immune reaction and the phenomenon of organ rejection. Limited also is its knowledge of tissue typing and the effect that a new heart may have on the mind. It has yet to develop an artificial organ whose materials are nontoxic and may be used without the danger of destroying the blood's chemistry. All these limitations taken together pose serious drawbacks for organ transplantation surgery at present. And yet, solutions for these problems are in the offing. Even these limitations will be lifted.

In addition to scientific and technological limitations medical science is confronted with another limitation that is peculiar in its nature. This limitation is neither scientific nor technological, but human. It involves, on the one hand, the need for viable transplant organs and, on the other hand, man's seeming inability to recognize the need.

The advent of organ transplantation surgery came as the dawn of a new day for thousands of patients suffering from incurable kidney and heart disease. The new day brought with it new hope. The victim of incurable kidney disease could be freed from the artificial kidney machine. The victim of incurable heart disease was given a final option.

Organ transplantation surgery has brought drama into the lives of those who suffer such incurable diseases. The drama itself, however, belongs to them and not to the man of sound body with normally functioning heart and kidneys. This man does not know the drama, because he has never been told that except for an organ transplant he would die. Such is the way of

human understanding that those who are of the world
of the living do not know what it is to be of the world
of the dying. It is the way of man that he truly under-
stands only that which he experiences in his own
body. A person may witness the suffering of a friend
who has incurable heart disease and see how limited
and pain-ridden that friend's life is, but a person with
a well heart does not suffer the disease nor the death
that is imminent, nor does he know what it is to need
a new heart.

A problem implicit in this day of organ transplantation surgery is that of organ procurement. There are
more people in need of organs than there are organs
available. Thousands of lives hang in the balance each
day, and the scales are weighted against the majority
of them because the demand exceeds the supply. The
suspense of the drama is paramount in cardiac transplantation surgery, where the life of one person depends upon the death of another. Life is precious to
someone who is about to lose it. On the other hand,
it is often taken for granted by those who have it
firmly within their grasp.

Some will find in this problem a religious dimension. For them the idea that out of the death of one
person can come life for another will be awe-inspir-
ing. Some will be able to see another's hope in the
misfortune of their loved one. Others will not. In
donating an organ in life or death, some will see the
fulfillment of the command: "Do unto others as you
would have them do unto you." How a person looks

upon this problem and whether or not he sees a religious dimension to it depends upon the feelings, temperament, and faith of the person involved.

Though the problem of organ procurement is a problem between human donors and human recipients, and thus is neither scientific nor technological in its nature, medical science is involved in it. In the past few years, medical science has been the champion of the cause of organ procurement.

The question of how the limitation is to be overcome (that is, how medical science is to procure organs) involves certain moral issues. The doctor has an obligation to the critically ill patient who is in need of a transplant. He is obligated to care for this patient as best he can within the situation. The physician, however, has a further obligation in regard to those whom he would wish to see as organ donors. Some there are who will recognize the great shortage of transplant organs and will decide to donate an organ. Others will recognize the need but will be unmoved by it. Still others will recognize the need and will stand in direct opposition to it. As sad, silly, and ironic as it will seem to some, the physician has obligations with respect to all these people. With what ease the problem would be solved if medical science had the right of removal at random of any or all of a man's organs at the time of his death! The question has been raised, however, by lay people and by members of the medical profession itself as to whether medical science does, in fact, have such a right.

What a task it is to respect the rights of man—to

respect his human rights, his political rights, his property rights. What a task, too, to respect his physical rights, the rights he has with regard to his own body. Is it not precisely here, in relation to a man's rights, that the question of the morality or the immorality of an issue or of an act is often focused?

Medical science, as a practice familiar with human needs and limitations, knows the need of man to be fed, to be kept warm, and to be cleansed. It knows the need of the injured to be relieved of pain and suffering. It knows the need of the sick to be made well. It knows the need of man to be understood no matter how irrational and jumbled his thoughts may seem to be. It knows that the man who today is unable to see the needs of the infirm and the dying is the same man who tomorrow may seek its help. It knows of man's seeming inability to be understanding, concerned, and compassionate regarding the needs of others. And yet, medical science knows of man beyond his momentary limitations and his shortcomings. It knows of man when he, so to speak, comes through. It knows the joy of a man who sees the needs of others and sets out to minister to those needs. It knows the joy of the man who gives to another something of himself not by force but by choosing to do so.

History records stories of men in battle who have given of themselves that others might live. Perhaps the closest thing to this in peaceful situations has been that of a man choosing to be used as an experimental subject in the hope that the knowledge gained will be of benefit in saving other lives. Now, with the dawn of organ transplantation surgery, man is shown another way to give. He may, by choosing to do so, give a part of himself as a gift of life to another. Medical science knows well that at present the only solution to the problem of the limited number of available transplant organs lies with the individual man and his willingness to give. It is to man and his willingness to give that medical science turns in the search for an answer to the problem of the present limitation.

The Problem of Organ Procurement

Organ transplantation surgery today has only two available organ graft sources, the living donor and the cadaver donor. Medical science has certain responsibilities to both of these sources.

The Living Donor. The living donor presents the medical practitioner with a number of special problems. One question that has arisen with regard to living donors is that of the nontherapeutic removal of an organ and whether or not it is a form of suicide for a person to seek the removal of an organ from his body that may save another person's life. The obvious reasoning behind this is that if an organ is so important that it could save the life of one person, will not the removal of it put in jeopardy the life of the donor?

Thoughts of suicide, partial self-destruction, and self-mutilation are distasteful for many people, to say the least. They may be regarded as not only distasteful but as morally reprehensible when one sees the physician as being partner to such acts. This is to be expected. The task of the physician is seen to be, on the one hand, that of preventing illness, and when prevention cannot be had, his task is seen to be therapeutic—to correct, to heal, to make well. To put in jeopardy the life of a healthy person through the removal of a healthy organ is then naturally seen to stand at odds with the physician's task even though the organ that is removed may save the life of another person.

The question of the moral reprehensibility of the acts of suicide and of partial self-destruction or self-mutilation is not new. Immanuel Kant, writing in the late eighteenth century, was familiar with these issues and the issue of the transplantation of bodily parts. According to the eighteenth-century philosopher, a man has certain duties to himself as an animal being. In his words, "The *first*, though not the highest, of man's duties to himself as an animal being is to preserve himself in his animal nature."[47] Animal nature, lest one become misled, may here be interpreted as man's physicality. Thus, Kant is saying that a man has the duty to himself to preserve his physical nature or to preserve himself physically. To commit suicide is, then, a wrong. Such an act constitutes the total destruction of man in his animal nature. Partial self-destruction or the mutilation of oneself, like suicide, is also seen to be a violation against oneself as an animal being. What lies behind the idea that a man has the duty to himself of preserving himself in his physical nature? Kant's concept of man is at issue here. For Kant a man is always a subject of duty. Man is himself the subject of morality. To cut one's life short or to endanger it knowingly is to "root out the existence of morality itself from the world, so far as that is in one's power."[48]

What meaning, if any, does this have for man and for medical science today? Kant's concept of man as the subject of morality and hence a subject of duty is no doubt alien to most people today. This is only natural. Such a philosophy cannot sit well in any age in which the morality or immorality of an act is seen to be virtually dependent upon the situation and the temper of the hearts and minds of those within the situation through whom the situation has its existence and gains its meaning. But even a time that is prone to see morality or immorality to be a matter of the situation stands to gain something from seeing the human body to be of importance and worth.

The human body has been and is a constant victim of all manner of degradation. Surely there has not been an age in recorded history when the human body has not been offended, assaulted, and degraded, be it by war or by other means. One need not wear the badge of a Kantian philosopher to respect the human body.

Medical science, as a science dedicated to the task of making man well and keeping him well, must necessarily hesitate to do anything to a man that would be in violation of his physical self. Surely the removal of a diseased organ cannot be seen to be such a violation. In fact, the removal of such an organ would contribute to the restoration of the man's physical self. What, however, of the removal of an organ that is not diseased, that is in fact well? What of the nontherapeutic removal of an organ? This is, of course, a question that is at hand in regard to the acceptance of organs from living donors. The removal of an organ from a living donor is not for the therapeutic benefit of that person. Is it, then, justified or justifiable?

The fact that the removal of an organ from a living donor is not for the donor's therapeutic benefit is not, morally speaking, the central issue. Whether or not the removal of an organ is therapeutic is a medical issue. The moral issue, and the issue central here, is whether or not the removal of an organ will jeopardize unduly the donor's physical being and existence. A science whose task it is to heal the injured and to make well the sick is duty bound to avoid the temptation to jeopardize the life of one person for the benefit of another.

The question of organ procurement is not merely the question of the need for a transplant organ on the part of the dying. The question necessarily goes beyond that of one man's need for an organ to the question of the possibility of endangering a second man's life through the removal of a healthy organ. The question that is naturally asked in regard to putting a second life in jeopardy is whether and how one knows that that life will, in fact, be put in peril. The physician does not always know what will happen to a person as a result of what is to be done to him. The unexpected is always possible. What the physician does not know in fact, however, he can and must postulate as a possibility. For him knowingly to jeopardize the life of a donor beyond a certain degree is without moral justification. To proceed to remove an organ not knowing in fact, but knowing that the possibility of endangering the life of the donor is great, is likewise morally unjustified. The practice of medicine, like the practice of government, finds itself from time to time in the peculiar situation in which the life of the one or the many can benefit from sacrificing another person or persons. Medical science, however, is not government. Though medical science knows of the ideology of the survival of the fittest, it does not guide itself by it. The physician shepherds the injured, the sick, and the dying that they may be healed, made well, and live. In his efforts to heal and to make well he must be cautious lest he destroy in order to save.

In refusing to do anything to a man (and here, in particular, to a prospective living donor) that would knowingly jeopardize his physical being and existence, the physician acts so as to affirm and foster a respect for the human body and for man's physical life, which is sorely needed today and at all times.

The physician's responsibility to the living donor does not end with the decision of whether or not the removal of an organ would put the donor's physical existence in peril. A large percentage of the donations from living donors are in the form of intrafamilial donations. That is, they are between twins—identical and nonidentical—between brothers and sisters, and between parents and children. A sad fact it is, and yet true, that there are families who see one family member or another to be of less value than the member who is dying and is in need of a transplant organ. Cases of pressuring the less valuable member to submit to donating an organ are not unknown. It is the doctor's responsibility to be aware of any such pressuring that would cause a person's willingness to be used as a living donor to come as the result of something other than his own free informed consent.

The idea of free informed consent, central to any justification in performing experimentations on human beings, is central also to the advisability and justification of accepting organs from living donors. The same issues regarding free informed consent are necessary here that are necessary in human experimentation. Any person who is under undue pressure, be it internal or external, is not capable of giving free consent. Likewise, any person who is intellectually unable to understand whatever risks may be involved or who is emotionally too unstable to handle the situation cannot give informed consent. Such consent thus depends upon the ability of the person to understand the risks involved and to be capable emotionally of withstanding the situation. Such a person must naturally be free of undue pressures if his consent is to be free. The guidelines and safeguards that have been set up with regard to human experimentation have an important part to play concerning the procurement of organs from living donors. The living

donor will always present the physician with certain
problems and questions. The question of the advisability and wisdom of the nontherapeutic removal of
organs from living donors is always warranted.

The Cadaver Donor. The bizarre fact that a possibility always exists that the living donor's life may
be put in jeopardy through the nontherapeutic removal of an organ puts medical science and the individual practitioner in a bind. Medical science and the
practitioner both know that a science whose task is
that of saving lives cannot, in its fervor to save lives,
be partner to the possible destruction of one life for
the benefit of another without arousing serious moral
questions. For this reason the cadaver donor is seen
by some to be medicine's best hope at present.

The American Medical Association and the American Bar Association have pledged themselves to an
act whose merit reflects the wisdom behind it. The
Uniform Anatomical Gift Act (the text of which is
included as an Appendix to this book) provides for
the right of any person, eighteen years of age and
older and of sound mind, to will in the form of a gift
his entire body or any part or parts of it after death
for the sake of research, transplantation, or for storage
in a tissue bank. The Act further provides that the
person's wishes cannot be overruled by the wishes of
the next of kin. Their wishes, however, may prevail in
the event that the person in question had not, in life,
exercised his right of deciding what would be done
with his body and parts after death.[49]

The merit of the Act is to be seen both in what it

provides and in what it avoids. Most importantly it avoids the issue of the buying and selling of organs in that it is a "gift" act. It likewise avoids the situation in which life becomes something to be had by the highest bidder.

The Uniform Anatomical Gift Act places the issue of organ donation firmly in the hands of the individual person. It is an act of the will, literally and metaphorically. A man enacts it in the form of a will and as a matter of his own free choice or desire to do so. It is of note that this Act does not give medical science the right of free postmortem removal of organs. In fact, the statement of the Act directly opposes this. This says something regarding medicine's respect for man and for his rights. Some there are, of course, who will uphold the issue of the postmortem at random removal of organs, contending that the need for organs is so great and that the remaining loved ones would never know the difference in that they do not care to inspect the body of the deceased. The reasoning holds true that the need for transplant organs is great and that the next of kin would not, under most circumstances, know the difference, but the fact is that the difference remains.

It may be true that the Act, which gives man the right to decide what medical science can and cannot do with his body and parts post-mortem, virtually assures that there will never be enough donor organs to fill the need. Sadly enough this already seems to be true. What is not saddening, however, is the fact that the Act illustrates medicine's belief that ends do

not always justify means regardless of how important
the ends are. Such an act affirms that not even the
great need that there is for viable transplant organs
justifies medicine's violation of what it sees to be a
man's rights.

Saving lives is important to medical science, and
yet it knows that how it goes about saving lives is
more important. The need for transplant organs is
great. Greater still, however, is the need for care as to
how those organs are to be procured. This age is
more than merely one in which medical science has
once again surpassed its own scientific and technological capabilities. It is an age in which medical
science has had to examine itself in terms of the rights
that a man has by the mere fact of his humanity.
Medical science knows very well how easily scientific
and technological advance can become negligent of a
man's human rights.

At times in the past, medical science has had to
take a stand for man and his human rights. At times,
no doubt, the stand that medicine arrived at seemed
to jeopardize its own hope for progress. Not so long
ago it had to take a stand regarding man and the
rights that a man has as an object of scientific investigation. Today medical science has taken a stand in
regard to the rights a man has to say what medical
science can do with his body after death. That medical science has had to examine itself in order to
understand what a man's rights are as a human being
is of benefit to man and is of no less benefit to medical
science itself.

Medical science has mastered the surgical technique necessary for organ transplantation surgery. What it has not mastered is the great need for transplant organs. It is safe to say that the need will not be met prior to the perfection of artificial organs. The Uniform Anatomical Gift Act is an attempt to understand and to grant to man those rights which are his simply because he is alive and is a human being. One of the limitations that medical science faces today is a human limitation. This is to say that it is a limitation between man and his fellowman. Such a limitation does not involve science and technology so much as it involves man's need to understand the needs and sufferings of others.

Recipient Selection

Medical science stands in a peculiar relationship to man. It stands not as the judge of his merits and worth but as a practice concerned lest his physical and psychological sufferings and needs destroy him. In an age which is so oriented to human accomplishments and a man's social worth that it is prone to see man only in these terms, it is refreshing to see in medical science a practice that is concerned for man and his sufferings. Such concern is not on the basis of any measure of his social worth or professional achievements, but it is due simply to the fact that he is alive and human, frail and of bodily needs. Few practices or endeavors see man in such terms.

The issue of recipient selection involves more than

simply the question of who will receive a transplant and who will not. Fundamentally the issue involves the question of the terms upon which medical science relates to those who seek its care.

It is quite evident that medical science and society as a whole relate to man in different terms. Society generally sees man in terms of his social worth and professional or nonprofessional station. It sees man not so much in terms of any potential he may have as in terms of what he overtly offers to society. This is to say that a man's social worth (or lack of it) is largely dependent upon his station, be it that of farmer, baker, candlestick maker, doctor, lawyer, or whatever. The man who offers the most to society in these social terms is seen to be of great worth, whereas the man whom society sees as overtly offering little or nothing (for example, the unemployed or the unemployable, regardless of whether they have or have not been given the chance and the right to offer something to society) is seen to be of lesser worth. Society, prone as it is to setting up value judgments, relates to man in terms of such judgments.

Medical science, on the other hand, though it recognizes man as a social being and thus as having social worth, relates to him in terms other than those of his social worth and professional station. This is to be expected. Medicine's task is not so much to see man in terms of what he offers to society as in terms of what his needs are. Medical science, as a practice that deals with man in his physical sufferings and needs, knows very well that disease, illness, and injury go beyond the artificial boundaries of class and station.

The science that is responsible to the sufferings of all finds itself today in the dilemma of choosing which few out of the many in need of organs will receive them. The question has been raised, with regard to recipient selection, as to the wisdom of implementing a standard for selection that is contrary to the terms upon which medical science relates to the sick and to the dying. The dilemma belongs to medical science; so too does the choosing. The dilemma is itself the question of whether medical science wishes to relate to man in terms of the humanity that all men share (and thus in terms of human suffering and need) or whether it wants to relate to him in terms of his worth to society.

Guidelines for Choosing. The purpose of organ transplantation surgery, be it the transplantation of the heart, kidney, lung, spleen, or whatever, is the long-term restoration of a critically ill patient to a productive and personally enjoyable life. To achieve this task the physician must utilize all the scientific genius and the technological skill available to him. The wise physician knows that, because of the nature and extent of their illnesses, not all critically ill patients can be so restored. Thus, the physician's task involves, in the first instance, determining who is medically qualified to receive a transplant.

The following points are suggested as guidelines for determining which patients are qualified from a strictly medical point of view. The phrase "qualified from a strictly medical point of view" means that the patient would have a reasonably good chance of being restored to a meaningful level of life.

First, the patient should be in critical need of a transplant organ. There should be no reasonable hope for his survival without the operation. This is of utmost importance when considering a patient for the transplant of a heart or for any other vital unpaired organ. Heart, liver, and spleen transplants are drastic both in their nature and in their outcome. Prognosis in the transplanting of vital unpaired organs has not been for long-term survival. It has often been for a year or less, with a physically painful and drug-dependent level of existence. At present the transplantation of vital unpaired organs should be recommended with extreme care, and only as a final option, until such time as the transplantation of such an organ can offer the probability of a return to a useful life for a number of years.

Ironically, and yet sensibly, though the patient should be critically ill to qualify for a transplant, he should not be so critically ill that he would not be likely to survive the transplant procedure. No matter how simple the surgical techniques may appear, the operation is heavy surgery for the patient to bear. Therefore, a second guideline is that the patient should at least enjoy enough overall physical well-being that he could physically and psychologically shoulder the burden.

Third, due consideration must be given to any complicating factors of the patient's condition. For example, critically ill heart patients often have serious ailments other than their cardiac condition, such as kidney or lung problems that could grossly complicate recovery. One would be warranted in questioning the wisdom of selecting a cardiac patient for a new heart if he were suffering from a chronic disease in addition to the cardiac problem.

Fourth, there must be due consideration of the disease that caused the destruction of the organ in the first place before the determination is made in respect to the transplant. That disease might, for example, be such as to destroy the transplant organ as well as the original one. The physician must be aware of any diseases that would indicate that the transplant should not be attempted.

These, then, are guidelines, not for selecting the recipients who will receive a transplant, but for determining whether a patient is medically qualified to be a potential candidate for transplantation. The actual procedure of and need for recipient selection arises ultimately because there will always be more patients qualified medically to receive organs than there will be organs available to meet the demand.

How does one proceed then with the task of selecting recipients? There are a number of possible ways. Suggested methods include selection by lot, by the highest success chance, by the age of the patient, and by the greatest value to medical science. Each of these approaches has its own merit.

Selection by lot would be impartial and unbiased. It could be instituted on a regional or on a nationwide scale. The available organ or organs could be rushed from one place to another once the recipient's name and hospital were made known.

Selection on the basis of the greatest chance of success merits consideration in that transplants are done in an attempt to provide successful treatment for patients with various critical illnesses. In view of this and of the fact that the supply cannot meet the demand, there is reason to consider a method of selection based on the issue of which few of the many would be most likely to experience the best results from the transplantations.

Recipient selection based upon the age of the patient operates on the generally justifiable rationale that the younger patient is more likely to survive a transplant and to return to a relatively enjoyable and meaningful level of life than would ordinarily be true of an older patient. Thus the slogan, "Bet on youth," is meaningful not only in the professional and business world; it is very timely and meaningful in regard to organ transplants.

Selection on the basis of which transplant would be of most value to medical science cannot be taken lightly. The physician has gained much knowledge and will gain more through transplanting organs as a research method and as a clinical trial. There have been times in the past and there will be times in the future when a transplant is highly unusual for one reason or another. The fact that medical science could gain important knowledge through transplantation in such an unusual case cannot easily be disre-

garded or discarded when the physician is faced with
the task of deciding who will and who will not receive a transplant. This final method of selection
always brings up the ticklish question of whether
medical science has an obligation to itself to further
its knowledge by utilizing the rare situation even
though it is certain that the attempt will offer little
or no benefit to the patient involved.

As can be seen, each of these suggested ways of
selecting recipients has something to offer. Though
each method has its merits, however, a person must
seriously question whether any one of them has
merit enough to justify it as the sole rationale for
selecting one individual over another to receive an
organ.

The lot method is artificial and disregards the
latest scientific developments, which ought not to be
overlooked in the selection process. Though the
method of selection based on the highest chance of
success is admirable and perhaps even in keeping
with the goal that transplant teams have set for themselves in performing operations, it seriously needs
interpretation lest one misinterpret the "success" of a
transplant to mean the mere prolongation of biological life. In the practice of medicine, success has
meant everything from the acquisition of knowledge
at the expense of the person, to the restoration of a
man's health and life, to the merciless act of prolonging a man's decline and process of dying.

The third suggested method of recipient selection
—on the basis of age—takes a very important factor

into consideration but to the exclusion of a number of other factors of no less importance. Among these are the patient's desire to withstand the operative procedure and its risks and his desire to be made well or whole again. It is granted that youth possesses a physical resiliency that is usually not present with the aging, but the wise physician knows that this is not always enough. Physical resiliency, in the absence of strength of mind and spirit, gives the physician little with which to work. Though the desire to stay alive is rarely of itself sufficient to save a person's life, crisis situations do develop during surgery and periods of postoperative care when such desire can mean the difference between a person's survival or death. One must remember that the desire to go on living is a mental attitude that is not necessarily relinquished with the decline of the physical self. In truth, the mental attitude may be sustained and strengthened as the body grows weaker. For these and other reasons, age alone is not a medically sound rationale for selecting one person instead of another as a recipient.

The fourth suggested method—selection on the basis of the greatest value to medical science—may have its place at times. The fact remains, however, that that which is of greatest value to the science of medicine as a whole is not necessarily of the most benefit to the patient in question. This is important because, though valuable knowledge may be gained in any transplant operation, transplants are supposedly being performed for the direct benefit of the patient who has been selected as a recipient. To perform a transplant under the guise of its being for the benefit of the recipient himself, when in fact it is being done purely or primarily for the purpose of acquiring knowledge, is an act of deceit. The physician who is party to it is to be held morally reprehensible.

What, however, one may ask, about the situation in which a critically ill patient volunteers to be used as an experimental subject, not on the basis of any possible benefit to himself but on the basis that the experiment might provide medical science with new knowledge? In the past, patients have been permitted to volunteer for experiments and have been accepted as experimental subjects for the testing of drugs and surgical procedures and techniques from which they could not receive direct benefit because of the nature and extent of their illnesses. Why then should a man not be permitted to volunteer for and be accepted as an experimental subject for an organ transplant performed for the explicit purpose of acquiring knowledge on the part of medical science?

No doubt this question bears heavily upon the minds of many physicians and many critically ill patients who are guided by a deep concern for the sufferings of others and who are aware that the knowledge gained through experimentation may be of value to others. The issue is difficult and cannot be dealt with, however, without considering a number of other important factors. One must consider these questions: How far is a man justified in using himself as a means? How far is he justified in permitting another person to use him as a means?

The transplantation of vital unpaired organs has in the past frequently indicated the imminence of the recipient's death. One must ask, therefore, if and under what circumstances a man is justified in using himself as a means to that extent. Of even greater importance is the question of how far patients and physicians are justified in using, for purely experimental purposes (the acquisition of knowledge), an organ that is in short supply when that usage will deprive another person of a chance at life.

Once again we are confronted by and unable to escape the question of what are the permissible limits of experimentation. What about experimentation and organ transplantation? At this point, a distinction needs to be made between "experimentation" and "experimental procedure." The transplantation of vital unpaired organs ought not to be a matter of experimentation. It is correctly seen to be an experimental procedure performed in the hope that it will serve as a method of treatment for the benefit of the recipient in his illness. The difference in purpose between experimentation and the use of an experimental procedure, then, is worth noting.

Experimentation represents an early stage in the quest for knowledge or skill. Its purpose is admittedly not the immediate benefit of the patient or subject. In experimentation, the patient or subject is, in fact, being used as a means of gaining the knowledge that is being sought. The orientation is not toward the present case but toward the future, toward the development of techniques or the acquisition of knowledge that will be used for the benefit of patients other than those subject to the experiment.

Experimentation involves moving toward or into relatively new fields of search and inquiry. The results of the experimentation may be anticipated, but they are not known. The purpose of experimentation is to discover what the results will be, to discover what the technique or procedure under consideration will actually accomplish. It is essential to note that in experimentation, service to the patient is secondary, while the quest for new knowledge is primary.

The purpose of transplanting a vital organ is not the same as that in experimentation. Such an operation ought not to be done for the sake of experimentation or for the sake of gaining pure knowledge. Experimentation as the search for knowledge is justified within reasonable limits, but one would need to question the morality of any attempt to gain knowledge when that attempt utilizes a procedure that is as drastic as the removal and replacement of a vital organ has proved to be.

Transplantation involving an unpaired organ ought not to be performed primarily for the purpose of experimentation. It ought not to be performed merely for the acquisition of knowledge. Considered from a moral point of view, such a transplant, because it is drastic both in nature and in outcome, ought to be attempted only on the basis that there is reason to believe such a procedure would be of benefit to the patient himself.

The transplantation of vital unpaired organs is properly called an experimental procedure because the element of certainty as to outcome is still relatively low, while the element of risk is relatively high. As a surgical procedure it is still in the stage of development or perfecting. It will be considered an experimental procedure by most physicians until such time as the risks and uncertainties involved in it are reduced to a degree warranting its acceptance as a "safe" clinical procedure.

The performance of this experimental procedure has afforded and will continue to afford the physician valuable knowledge. In purpose, however, it will continue to differ from experimentation in that, though knowledge may be gained, the knowledge gained is incidental to the primary goal of the procedure, which is to provide treatment for the patient.

What, then, does this have to say regarding or in reply to the suggested method of selecting recipients on the basis of the greatest value to medical science? In the first place, it needs to be noted that that which is of greatest value to medical science may be seen to stand at odds with what has been stated as the purpose of organ transplantation surgery. Though the purpose of medical science is the promotion of human well-being, it is the acquisition of knowledge that is often considered to be of greatest value.

In the second place, considering the fact that the purpose of an organ transplant (and consequently that which is of greatest value in the transplant) is to provide treatment for the patient and is not for the acquisition of knowledge, a conflict of values arises. To the extent that what is of greatest value to medical science is not consistent with the attempt to benefit the patient directly by means of a transplant attempt, it seems highly unwise and unfitting to employ this as the criterion of selection. This is to imply, of course, that the criterion used for selecting recipients should be in keeping with the purpose of the transplant itself. What is needed is a method of selection that can offer the best possible assurance that the transplant recipient may benefit significantly from the operation. This calls for a medically sound method, one that takes into consideration the latest developments and discoveries of transplant research. It calls also for a morally sound method, one that takes into consideration the rights and the dignity of the patient, that sees him not merely as a subject for experimentation but as a fully human person.

Tissue Matching and Typing. Research over the past few years has provided the physician with two medically sound procedures that are being used in the selection of organ transplant recipients by various medical centers throughout the world. Experience has shown both the researcher and the transplanter that the better the tissue match between donor and recipient, the greater the chance of the transplant's survival. The meaning and importance of this are not to be overlooked. Tissue matching provides a medically sound and morally justifiable rationale for choosing one patient over another for an organ transplant. It is medically sound in that there is very strong reason to believe that " 'when a donor is unrelated, selection of the recipient on the basis of the tissue match can improve the prognosis.' "[50] It is morally justified in that benefit to the patient is of utmost importance.

The idea of tissue matching arose out of a natural sequence of events. The pioneers of organ transplantation realized that transplants between identical twins were less likely to undergo a rejection reaction than were transplants between other related persons. They also realized that transplants between nonidentical siblings were less likely to be rejected than were transplants between a donor and a recipient chosen at random. This realization raised the issue of tissue compatibility, and researchers began to ask whether by typing and matching the tissues of unrelated donors and recipients the probability of severe organ rejection might be reduced and thus the results of transplants between unrelated persons might become similar to the results of transplants between related donors and recipients. The question involved a gamble, but some researchers felt that it offered a chance. Today, many physicians feel that the techniques developed by those scientists offer the greatest hope for the future success of organ transplants between unrelated donors.

Two processes are involved here—tissue matching and tissue typing. The process of matching tissues relies upon the technique referred to as tissue typing.

This, as the name implies, involves typing or classifying tissues according to their leukocyte antigens. The technique is somewhat analogous to typing blood. The major difference between the two techniques is that the substances of which the pathologist makes the type are different. In typing blood, the pathologist types cell to sera and sera to cell, whereas in typing tissues he is typing the antigens of the white cells.

Overlooking the differences of the techniques, however, their purpose is the same. For example, blood is typed so that in blood transfusions (or "blood transplants") the physician will know the proper type of blood to use. A person with A-negative blood, in need of a transfusion, would be given A-negative blood or a blood type compatible with it. In like manner, typing is done on tissues to ensure that a suitable donor-recipient tissue combination may be obtained. By "suitable donor-recipient tissue combination" is meant a tissue match whereby the donor tissue is compatible with the tissues of the recipient. Tissue matching, then, in fact, involves matching the available organ to the proper recipient according to tissue type.

The process of matching a donor organ with the proper recipient may be likened to the task of a seamstress in matching plaids. Anyone who sews knows that there are many different plaids and that plaids vary by pattern and color. Identical plaids can be worked together into a perfect match. Nonidentical plaids, on the other hand, cannot be made to produce a perfect match, but some nonidentical plaids can be worked together to give a suitable match. Other plaids, however, vary so in pattern and color that they are completely incompatible when brought together. They are utterly incapable of existing together in harmony because their patterns do not agree in any way.

Between the identical plaids, which offer a perfect match, and the plaids that are a total mismatch, there are plaids that offer varying degrees of compatibility. The seamstress, looking for a perfect match, would naturally look for identical plaids. Unable to find them, but wanting to have a near-perfect match, she would look for the plaids that would be most compatible. Similarly, utilizing the tissue-matching technique, the transplant surgeon would look for a recipient identical in tissue type to the donor's tissue type. If he could not find an identical match, he would look for a donor-recipient combination as nearly identical or compatible as possible.

Tissue-typing Programs. One of the finest examples of the use of tissue-typing techniques and tissue matching as a means of selecting organ recipients is the Eurotransplant program. This is an international organ-exchange program that utilizes the tissue-typing methods developed in the United States by Dr. Paul I. Terasaki. Twenty-eight medical centers participate in this five-nation program.

Under the program, recipients are typed before donor organs are available. The information regarding the recipient's tissue type is fed into a computer along with other facts about the patient, such as age, sex, blood type, and state of his disease. Recipient lists are updated and distributed at least once a month to the various tissue-typing centers in the program.

When a hospital in the program has a prospective donor, it gets in contact with the nearest tissue-typing center. Within a few hours the typing center notifies the hospital regarding the donor's test results and supplies the hospital with the names and addresses of the most likely recipients. The decision as to who will receive the organ is not made by the typing center. The center merely types the tissues and makes the pertinent information available. The decision as to whether the organ is accepted for use is made by the recipient's physician. The matter of transferring the organ is handled by the hospitals of the donor and the recipient.

It is of note that the success of this program, or of any program like it, depends in large part upon the number of prospective recipient participants. In the words of Dr. J. J. Van Rood, one of Eurotransplant's organizers, to obtain the best donor-recipient combination it is necessary "to have a large number of potential recipients, representing a broad spectrum of antigen combinations with which to match your donor."[51]

Programs similar to the European program have taken shape in the United States. There is the National Transplant Registry in Boston; and computer

matching services for organ donors and recipients
have been established in Chicago and Los Angeles.
These programs are mainly geared to kidney transplants, but they are also matching for transplants of
vital unpaired organs, including hearts and spleens.
Again, the success of these programs, like that of the
European program, depends largely upon the number
of participating hospitals and recipients. The reason
for this is obvious. The more recipients there are to
choose from, the greater the chances for a near-
perfect tissue match.

Concluding Observations. A few observations may
be made, finally, regarding tissue matching as a
rationale for selecting the few, out of the many in
need of organs, who will receive them. In the first
instance, tissue matching as a method of selection is
consistent with the purpose of medical science—the
promotion of human well-being. Just what constitutes
the promotion of human well-being in any case, however, is not always possible to predict.

There may be times when, because of an ideal or a
good tissue match between the donor and the recipient, the patient's overall well-being may be promoted
by a transplant. Experience in the past, however, has
indicated that when the tissue match between the
donor and the recipient was only fair or poor, the
patient generally underwent a furious rejection reaction, with psychological abnormalities developing in
some cases, and resultant death.

By means of tissue typing and tissue matching, the

physician may know in advance whether the patient would be likely to benefit and whether it would be wise to perform the transplant. These methods would also tell him that beyond a certain acceptable degree of mismatch a transplant ought not to be performed.

In the second instance, tissue matching can help the physician determine how and where an available organ can best be used. Man has throughout history tolerated and been party to the waste of nonvaluable materials and of valuable materials that were in abundance. Responsible men, however, ought not to and must not tolerate the waste of valuable and scarce materials of which another is in dire need. What few human organs there are available for transplanting are precious beyond words. Such precious material ought not to be used indiscriminately. Tissue matching offers a method of using tissues discriminatively, not on the basis of a man's skin color, brain, or beliefs, but rather on the basis of his tissue type and need. It thus provides a means of assuring that the few organs available will be used in those transplant attempts which are most likely to succeed because of a good match, thereby promoting the well-being of the person involved.

A third, but no less important, observation is that tissue matching offers a means of recipient selection that is in keeping with the terms upon which medical science relates to man. Research done in the area of organ transplantation surgery (including tissue typing and tissue matching) takes into consideration and is involved with the person in his sickness and in his need, regardless of his professional or nonprofessional station in life.

The importance of thus implementing a method of selecting recipients that is consistent with the terms upon which medical science relates to man ought not to be forgotten. Though medical science is well aware of human potential and strength, it is also aware that injury, illness, and disease can render man frail of body and great of need. Transplantation research recognizes man's frailty and need and is providing ways of coping with these. Tissue matching as a method of recipient selection takes medical science and the physician one more step along the way toward relieving human suffering caused by certain as yet incurable diseases.

Organ Transplantation: Retrospect and Prospect

THE SHAPE OF TOMORROW

As medical science stands in anticipation of tomorrow, it has placed upon it the task that confronts any man and any science which would stand responsibly on the brink of new beginnings. The task is to have vision, retrospective and prospective—to look back and to look forward. Whence has medical science come that it is this day where it is? What have been its discoveries that its burdens and successes are what they are? What has it not mastered that its limitations are as they are? What does the present hold in store for the future, or are the two disjointed and unconnected? Is today merely the day that stands between yesterday and tomorrow, merely a day that separates the two, or is it today that integrates the two and gives tomorrow its shape?

Medicine will go tomorrow where it will go because of where it has been and where it is today. The man who comes to this day unconcerned with the events and the happenings that brought him to this day and

brought this day to him faces the prospect of a shape-
less and, in that respect, meaningless and empty
future. The same holds true of medical science. Medical science cannot decree what tomorrow will bring,
but it can decree what it intends the future to be and
to hold and the part it wishes to play in that future.

In decreeing what it wants the future to be and to
hold in store, medical science does not decree for a
future that will involve itself alone. The field of medical science, like the field of politics, is in essence
people. My world, like your world, is shaped by the
decisions that medical science makes.

It is the duty of the medical scientist today to
decide about tomorrow. To go blindly into tomorrow
is without excuse for a science whose future looms so
great. For a man to go blindly into tomorrow is for
him to do wrong to all that and to all those who
depend upon him and upon what he does in the
future. For medical science to go blindly into tomorrow is for it to do wrong to all those for whom it exists.
Vision, retrospective and prospective, is medicine's
only defense against its own blindness.

Looking Back

Just yesterday medical science mastered the surgical technique necessary for the transplantation of
organs from one person to another. The minds that
conceived and made actual the renal transplantation
surgical technique made medical science heir to the
challenge of transplanting any vital organ. In the past

fifteen years or so, medical science has taken up the challenge. To date, transplantation attempts have been made for most of the body's vital organs—lung, liver, and heart included. In regard to the liver and the heart, the attempts have been drastic both in their nature and in their outcome. Drastic in nature because each of these is a vital unpaired organ. Drastic in outcome because the attempts have proved to be relatively unsuccessful in terms of patient recovery to an active and meaningful level of life.

There is no questioning the need for organ transplantation surgery. The number of deaths that are caused each year by irreparably damaged and diseased organs testifies to the need. And yet, in looking back, one realizes that the temptation has arisen to see organ transplantation as being all-important. In realizing the time and energy that have been spent on it in the past few years, the need becomes evident for keeping this phenomenon of medical advance in perspective. Organ transplantation surgery is important, but it is not all-important. Nothing is all-important to medical science save the promotion of human well-being and the manner in which medical science goes about doing this. Organ transplantation surgery is one means to this end, but it is not the only means. One should realize that the need for medical science to be so caught up in the task of healing and making well has come about, in part, because it has not yet fully realized (and therefore has not accomplished) the most basic of its tasks—that of disease prevention.

As harsh as it may seem to some, any decision made

today regarding the transplantation of vital unpaired organs in the future must be tempered with the wisdom that such a surgical technique will be of benefit to but a limited few. To say that medicine's ultimate concern should always be that of disease prevention, because such prevention will benefit the many, must not be misinterpreted to read that those for whom the transplantation of vital organs would be beneficial are not of importance to medical science. This is not the case. The conscience of medical science bears heavily the burden of the suffering and the need of those anxious for a transplant, but at the same time, it knows that the only way to get ahead of such suffering and need is through preventing the diseases that cause the suffering and need in the first place.

Looking back some twenty years or so, we may remember that medical science had much to rejoice over in the development and perfection of the iron lung, the rocking bed, and walking braces as a means to restoring the child with infantile paralysis to a meaningful level of life. Greater still, however, we remember the joy that came through the development of the vaccine that stands to this day as a preventive against polio. There is no doubting the need that there was for the iron lung and the rocking bed, but the fact that they were necessary made even more necessary a preventive for the disease that begged their development.

Such a situation is analogous to the situation that medical science faces in regard to organ transplantation surgery. Surgery such as this is necessary today and will be necessary in the future just as the iron lung was necessary in the past and, in some cases, is still necessary. The necessity for organ transplantation surgery, like the necessity for the iron lung, however, arose out of the presence of disease. The need for spending time and genius on disease prevention must not be lost in the midst of the excitement and the turmoil created by medicine's most recent scientific and technological advance.

It is often said that a man's hindsight is greater than his foresight. History has proved this again and again. The unwise publicity that has surrounded the transplantation attempts has served to sensationalize medicine's achievement and to arouse and then to dull human hope. Hope is a thing precious to all, the healthy and the sick alike, but more dear still is it to the dying patient who has little or no hope. Granted, the dying person often holds to one sort of hope or another. One may hold fast to the hope that his death will be painless and quick. Another man may cherish the hope that his loved ones will be at his side at the time of his passing. The hope to go on living through an organ transplantation, however, is a hope that in the past was actually open to but a few victims of incurable heart disease. Such a lack of hope was due partly to the shortage of available transplant organs and to the fact that the degenerate condition of many cardiac disease victims made surgery impossible. It was just such a hope as this, the hope of life, which was unwisely sold to the public and which the public in turn bought.

Some members of the medical profession have already spoken of the tragedy of the publicity that has surrounded the cardiac transplantation attempts. It is the news media's desire to get the story quickly and to sell it to the public, but medical science has paid a high price for such quickness and salability. Word of the transplants reached the public before it even reached professional colleagues. The information that needed first to be shared and evaluated at a professional level was made public property. What belonged to medical genius and to a few whom it could benefit at the moment was sold to an audience lacking the criteria and the tools with which to deal with it.

There is no questioning that the public has a right to know about the advances made by medical science, but the public has also the need to see such medical advances both in perspective and as they really are. Selling false hope, instilling hope where there was no hope, building up hope in persons for whom little hope existed is part of the price that has been paid today by an age that has taken to itself what does not yet fully belong to it and is not yet fully its own to enjoy. Organ transplantation surgery has a part to play in the future and is part of the shape of the future. Hopefully it has not been seriously jeopardized by the publicity that has surrounded it.

Cardiac transplantation surgery began only two years ago. To January, 1970, there were 154 transplants, with 24 survivors. It would be unfair to evaluate cardiac transplantations on the basis of the figures alone, and yet the figures speak of a need for continual evaluation and reevaluation. In terms of the number of survivors, the statistics betray a relatively unsuccessful procedure. It is safe to say that any new drug instrumental to such a drastic mortality rate would be withdrawn immediately. The same holds true for any car on the highway or plane in the sky. There is a difference here, however, and it begs realization. Cardiac transplants are performed only on those critically ill patients for whom the prognosis without a transplant is that of impending death within a few weeks or months. For such patients the transplants are but a final hope—the only available option. (Though the probability that the patient would have died anyway is in itself no justification for the continuation of a procedure that has proved to be so unsuccessful numberwise, the truth of the statement must be realized and accepted.)

Perhaps the best way at present to evaluate cardiac transplantation surgery is to approach it in terms of the quality of life it gives to the patient who survives rather than in terms of the number who survive. For such an evaluation one must turn to the records of those who have survived. Of the 24 survivors, one must ask whether they have been given a meaningful level of life or merely a prolonged state of suffering and need. Has their well-being been served or has their agony and process of dying merely been continued? If cardiac transplantation surgery is at present justified, its justification is on the criterion that it has served to promote human well-being. Once again the promotion of human well-being is seen to be both medicine's purpose and its dilemma.

In looking at organ transplantation in retrospect, one sees both the need for it and also some of the mistakes that have been made regarding it. Hopefully such retrospective vision will be of benefit to medical science as it looks forward.

LOOKING FORWARD

Medicine is a powerful science. Powerful, not in the sense of brute physical force, but in the sense of intellect and genius. It is the responsibility of medical science today to sit down with the power it has and endeavor to understand the force and potential of its power. If medical science has the power to build up, it also has the power to tear down. If it has the power to create, so too does it have the power to destroy. Power that is so glorious today can tomorrow be power demonic. Being destructive and being destroyed are the risks of having power and being powerful, but destroying and being destroyed need not be the ultimate end of power. Whether the power that medical science has today will be power glorious or power demonic depends upon how it utilizes its knowledge in overt actions.

Knowledge not parented by wisdom is but an illegitimate child of the intellect, susceptible to misdirection and misuse. Medical science needs the wisdom of foresight to know where it is going with the

decisions that it makes today. As a result of yesterday's accomplishments, the possibility of brain transplants and of genetic control loom in the future. What
of man and the world, however, when such possibilities become an accomplished fact? Will man and the
world be better off for what the scientist's knowledge
will enable him to do? The answer to this cannot be,
"Wait and see." Most of our moral dilemmas come as
a result of our inability to see where what we are
doing is taking us.

Before tomorrow comes, with all its potential,
promise, and hope, there is the need to realize that
the science which may have the ability to transplant
the human brain and control a man's intellect and
emotions could likewise have the ability to alter the
course of human life—its drives, appreciations, and
sensitivities. Ponder for a moment a world in which
parents could choose the intellectual level of their
unborn child. Then ponder the situation of the child
of average intelligence born into a world in which his
parents could have chosen otherwise. To be average
or below average in a world in which averageness or
below averageness was not of one's own choosing is
one thing. Man has a way of tolerating and even
accepting and loving that which could be none other
than it is, but to tolerate, let alone accept or love,
what could have been different through choice is
quite another task.

The time to ask whether or not man would want to
live in such a world is now, before that world is an
accomplished fact. The thought of being able to

determine a child's coloring, build, and intelligence level before birth is great and terrible at the same time. Great in the sense of the genius that made it possible, terrible in the sense that not all who will be capable of doing it will be wise enough to know whether it ought in fact to be done.

Today is the age of organ transplantation surgery. Tomorrow will be the age of genetic control. The way in which medical science uses its power (that is to say, how medical science utilizes its knowledge in overt actions) today will help to shape the future of man. Medical science is under obligation to stand responsibly before God and man today and always in order that its power tomorrow will be power glorious.

Appendix
Uniform Anatomical Gift Act

The Uniform Anatomical Gift Act was drafted by the National Conference of Commissioners on Uniform State Laws. At its Annual Conference Meeting in Philadelphia, Pennsylvania, July 22 through August 1, 1968, the Commissioners approved and recommended the Act for enactment in all the states. The proposed Act was approved by the American Bar Association at its meeting in Philadelphia, Pennsylvania, on August 7, 1968, and by the American Medical Association's House of Delegates at its meeting in Miami Beach, Florida, in December, 1968. A majority of the states have enacted legislation based on the Act, but with modifications in some instances. The text of the Uniform Anatomical Gift Act follows.

UNIFORM ANATOMICAL GIFT ACT

An act authorizing the gift of all or part of a human body after death for specified purposes.

SECTION 1. [*Definitions.*]
(a) "Bank or storage facility" means a facility licensed, accredited, or approved under the laws of any state for storage of human bodies or parts thereof.

(b) "Decedent" means a deceased individual and includes a stillborn infant or fetus.

(c) "Donor" means an individual who makes a gift of all or part of his body.

(d) "Hospital" means a hospital licensed, accredited, or approved under the laws of any state; includes a hospital operated by the United States government, a state, or a subdivision thereof, although not required to be licensed under state laws.

(e) "Part" means organs, tissues, eyes, bones, arteries, blood, other fluids and any other portions of a human body.

(f) "Person" means an individual, corporation, government or governmental subdivision or agency, business trust, estate, trust, partnership or association, or any other legal entity.

(g) "Physician" or "surgeon" means a physician or surgeon licensed or authorized to practice under the laws of any state.

(h) "State" includes any state, district, commonwealth, territory, insular possession, and any other area subject to the legislative authority of the United States of America.

SECTION 2. [*Persons Who May Execute an Anatomical Gift.*]

(a) Any individual of sound mind and 18 years of age or more may give all or any part of his body for any purpose specified in Section 3, the gift to take effect upon death.

(b) Any of the following persons, in order of priority stated, when persons in prior classes are not available at the time of death, and in the absence of actual notice of contrary indications by the decedent or actual notice of opposition by a member of the same or a prior class, may give all or any part of the decedent's body for any purpose specified in Section 3:

(1) the spouse,
(2) an adult son or daughter,
(3) either parent,
(4) an adult brother or sister,
(5) a guardian of the person of the decedent at the time of his death,
(6) any other person authorized or under obligation to dispose of the body.

(c) If the donee has actual notice of contrary indications by the decedent or that a gift by a member of a class is opposed by a member of the same or a prior class, the donee shall not accept the gift. The persons authorized by subsection (b) may make the gift after or immediately before death.

(d) A gift of all or part of a body authorizes any examination necessary to assure medical acceptability of the gift for the purposes intended.

(e) The rights of the donee created by the gift are paramount to the rights of others except as provided by Section 7 (d).

SECTION 3. [*Persons Who May Become Donees; Purposes for Which Anatomical Gifts May Be Made.*] The following persons may become donees of gifts of bodies or parts thereof for the purposes stated:

(1) any hospital, surgeon, or physician, for medical or dental education, research, advancement of medical or dental science, therapy, or transplantation; or
(2) any accredited medical or dental school, college or university for education, research, advancement of medical or dental science, or therapy; or
(3) any bank or storage facility, for medical or dental education, research, advancement of medical or dental science, therapy, or transplantation; or

(4) any specified individual for therapy or tranplantation needed by him.

SECTION 4. [*Manner of Executing Anatomical Gifts.*]

(a) A gift of all or part of the body under Section 2 (a) may be made by will. The gift becomes effective upon the death of the testator without waiting for probate. If the will is not probated, or if it is declared invalid for testamentary purposes, the gift, to the extent that it has been acted upon in good faith, is nevertheless valid and effective.

(b) A gift of all or part of the body under Section 2 (a) may also be made by document other than a will. The gift becomes effective upon the death of the donor. The document, which may be a card designed to be carried on the person, must be signed by the donor in the presence of 2 witnesses who must sign the document in his presence. If the donor cannot sign, the document may be signed for him at his direction and in his presence in the presence of 2 witnesses who must sign the document in his presence. Delivery of the document of gift during the donor's lifetime is not necessary to make the gift valid.

(c) The gift may be made to a specified donee or without specifying a donee. If the latter, the gift may be accepted by the attending physician as donee upon or following death. If the gift is made to a specified donee who is not available at the time and place of death, the attending physician upon or following death, in the absence of any expressed indication that the donor desired otherwise, may accept the gift as donee. The physician who becomes a donee under this subsection shall not participate in the procedures for removing or transplanting a part.

(d) Notwithstanding Section 7 (b), the donor may designate in his will, card, or other document of gift the surgeon or physician to carry out the appropriate procedures. In the absence of a designation or if the designee is not available, the donee or other person authorized to accept the gift may employ or authorize any surgeon or physician for the purpose.

(e) Any gift by a person designated in Section 2 (b) shall be made by a document signed by him or made by his telegraphic recorded telephonic, or other recorded message.

SECTION 5. [*Delivery of Document of Gift.*] If the gift is made by the donor to a specified donee, the will, card, or other document, or an executed copy thereof, may be delivered to the donee to expedite the appropriate procedures immediately after death. Delivery is not necessary to the validity of the gift. The will, card, or other document, or an executed copy thereof, may be deposited in any hospital, bank or storage facility or registry office that accepts it for safekeeping or for facilitation of procedures after death. On request of any interested party upon or after the donor's death, the person in possession shall produce the document for examination.

SECTION 6. [*Amendment or Revocation of the Gift.*] (a) If the will, card, or other document or executed copy thereof, has been delivered to a specified donee, the donor may amend or revoke the gift by:

(1) the execution and delivery to the donee of a signed statement, or

(2) an oral statement made in the presence of 2 persons and communicated to the donee, or

(3) a statement during a terminal illness or injury addressed to an attending physician and communicated to the donee, or

(4) a signed card or document found on his person or in his effects.

(b) Any document of gift which has not been delivered to the donee may be revoked by the donor in the manner set out in subsection (a), or by destruction, cancellation, or mutilation of the document and all executed copies thereof.

(c) Any gift made by a will may also be amended or revoked in the manner provided for amendment or revocation of wills, or as provided in subsection (a).

SECTION 7. [*Rights and Duties at Death.*]

(a) The donee may accept or reject the gift. If the donee accepts a gift of the entire body, he may, subject to the terms of the gift, authorize embalming and the use of the body in funeral services. If the gift is of a part of the body, the donee, upon the death of the donor and prior to embalming, shall cause the part to be removed without unnecessary mutilation. After removal of the part, custody of the remainder of the body vests in the surviving spouse, next of kin, or other persons under obligation to dispose of the body.

(b) The time of death shall be determined by a physician who tends the donor at his death, or, if none, the physician who certifies the death. The physician shall not participate in the procedures for removing or transplanting a part.

(c) A person who acts in good faith in accord with the terms of this Act or with the anatomical gift laws of another state [or a foreign country] is not liable for damages in any civil action or subject to prosecution in any criminal proceeding for his act.

(d) The provisions of this Act are subject to the laws of this state prescribing powers and duties with respect to autopsies.

SECTION 8. [*Uniformity of Interpretation.*] This Act shall be so construed as to effectuate its general purpose to make uniform the law of those states which enact it.

SECTION 9. [*Short Title.*] This Act may be cited as the Univorm [sic] Anatomical Gift Act.

SECTION 10. [*Repeal.*] The following acts and parts of acts are repealed:
(1)
(2)
(3)

SECTION 11. [*Time of Taking Effect.*] This Act shall take effect . . . . .

Notes

1. Frank J. Ayd, "What Is Death?" Unpublished article presented at the Second National Congress on Medical Ethics, sponsored by the Judicial Council of the American Medical Association, Chicago, Ill., Oct. 5–6, 1968, p. 2.

2. Theodore Fox, "Purposes of Medicine," *Lancet*, Vol. 2 (1965), p. 801; quoted by Ayd, "What Is Death?" p. 7.

3. Ayd, "What Is Death?" p. 14.

4. Immanuel Kant, *Foundations of the Metaphysics of Morals*, tr. by Lewis White Beck (The Bobbs-Merrill Company, Inc., 1965), p. 47.

5. G. E. Schreiner, in *Ethics in Medical Progress*, ed. by G. E. W. Wolstenholme and Maeve O'Connor (Little, Brown and Company, 1966), p. 74. (Hereafter referred to as *Ethics in Medical Progress*.)

6. Samuel Enoch Stumpf, "The Changing Mores of Biomedical Research," *Annals of Internal Medicine*, Vol. 67, No. 3, Part 2, Supplement 7 (Sept., 1967), p. 11.

7. *Ibid.*

8. *Ibid.*, p. 12.

9. *Ibid.*, pp. 13–14.

10. "After 25 Centuries, 1968 Became 'The Year of Transplants,'" *Journal of the American Medical Associa-*

tion, Vol. 206, No. 13 (Dec. 23–30, 1968), p. 2835. (Hereafter cited as "After 25 Centuries.") (Later references to the *Journal* will be cited as *JAMA.*)

11. Francis D. Moore *et al.,* "Cardiac and Other Organ Transplantation," *JAMA,* Vol. 206, No. 11 (Dec. 9, 1968), pp. 2489–2490. (Hereafter cited as "Cardiac and Other.")

12. *Ibid.,* p. 2490.

13. Helen B. Taussig, "A Time for Waiting," *The Johns Hopkins Magazine,* Spring, 1969, p. 9.

14. *Ethics in Medical Progress,* p. 57.

15. *Ibid.*

16. "Status of Transplantation 1968," A Report by the Surgery Training Committee of the National Institute of General Medical Sciences, National Institutes of Health, Bethesda, Md., Nov., 1968 (unpublished), p. 8.

17. "After 25 Centuries," p. 2834.

18. "Status of Transplantation 1968," p. 9.

19. *Ethics in Medical Progress,* p. 104.

20. "Status of Transplantation 1968," pp. 43–44.

21. Taussig, "A Time for Waiting," p. 11.

22. "Cardiac and Other," p. 2493.

23. Cf. "Psychiatric Effects in Organ Transplants," *Modern Medicine,* June 30, 1969, p. 23.

24. Cf. "What Does a New Heart Do to the Mind?" *Medical World News,* May 23, 1969, p. 17.

25. *Ibid.,* pp. 17–18.

26. Taussig, "A Time for Waiting," p. 11.

27. Editorial, "What and When Is Death?" *JAMA,* Vol. 204, No. 6, (May 6, 1968), p. 220.

28. Ayd, "What Is Death?" p. 2.

29. *Ibid.*

30. *Ibid.*

31. *Ibid.,* pp. 5–6.

32. *Ibid.,* p. 2.

33. *Ibid.*

34. *Ibid.,* p. 3.

35. Leonard Stevens, "What Is Death?" *Reader's Digest*, Vol. 94, No. 565 (May, 1969), pp. 225–232.

36. Cf. Ayd, "What Is Death?", p. 3.

37. Paul Ramsey, "On Updating Death," in *The Religious Situation 1969*, ed. by Donald Cutler (Beacon Press, Inc., 1969), 2d in a series of annual volumes, p. 257.

38. Ad Hoc Committee of the Harvard Medical School, "A Definition of Irreversible Coma," *JAMA*, Vol. 205, No. 6 (Aug. 5, 1968).

39. *Ibid.*, pp. 337–338.

40. *Ibid.*

41. *Ibid.*

42. *Ibid.*, p. 338.

43. Vincent J. Collins, "Limits of Medical Responsibility in Prolonging Life," *JAMA*, Vol. 206, No. 2 (Oct. 7, 1968), p. 391.

44. Ramsey, in Cutler (ed.), *op. cit.*, p. 268.

45. *Ibid.*, p. 269.

46. *Ibid.*

47. Immanuel Kant, *The Doctrine of Virtue*, tr. by Mary J. Gregor (Harper & Row, Publishers, Inc., 1964), p. 84.

48. *Ibid.*, p. 85.

49. "Transplant Rounds," *Medical World News*, July 11, 1969, p. 21.

50. "Rushing Donor Organs Across Europe's Borders," *Medical World News*, July 18, 1969, pp. 28–29.

51. *Ibid.*, pp. 30–31.

Selected Bibliography

BOOKS

Blaiberg, Philip, *Looking at My Heart*. Stein and Day, 1968.

Cutler, Donald (ed.), *The Religious Situation 1969*. Beacon Press, Inc., 1969.

Edmunds, Vincent, and Scorer, Gordon (eds.), *Ideals in Medicine: A Christian Approach to Medical Practice*. London: Tyndale Press, 1958.

Freund, Paul A., *et al.*, "Ethical Aspects of Experimentation with Human Subjects," *Daedalus*, Spring, 1969.

Hawthorne, Peter, *The Transplanted Heart*. Rand McNally & Company, 1968.

Jackson, D. M., *Medical Ethics and Morality*. London: Tyndale Press, 1958.

Kant, Immanuel, *The Doctrine of Virtue*, tr. by Mary J. Gregor. Harper & Row, Publishers, Inc., 1964.

———— *Foundations of the Metaphysics of Morals*, tr. by Lewis White Beck. The Bobbs-Merrill Company, Inc., 1965.

Ladimer, Irving, and Newman, Roger W. (eds.), *Clinical Investigation in Medicine: Legal, Ethical and Moral Aspects*. Boston University Law-Medicine Research Institute, 1963.

Moore, F. D., *Give and Take: The Development of Tissue Transplantations*. W. B. Saunders Company, 1964.

O'Connor, Maeve, and Wolstenholme, G. E. W. (eds.), *Ethics in Medical Progress*. Little, Brown and Company, 1966.

Snow, C. P., *The Two Cultures and the Scientific Revolution*, 2d ed. Cambridge University Press, 1964.

Tournier, Paul, *The Meaning of Persons*. Harper and Brothers, 1957.

Weber, Hans-Ruedi (ed.), *Experiments with Man*. (World Council of Churches Studies No. 6), World Council of Churches and Friendship Press, 1969.

White, Dale (ed.), *Dialogues in Medicine and Theology*. Abingdon Press, 1968.

PERIODICALS

Ad Hoc Committee of the Harvard Medical School, "A Definition of Irreversible Coma," *JAMA*, Vol. 205, No. 6 (Aug. 5, 1968), pp. 337–340.

"After 25 Centuries, 1968 Became 'The Year of Transplants,'" *JAMA*, Vol. 206, No. 13 (Dec. 23–30, 1968), pp. 2834–2835.

Alexander, S., "They Decide Who Lives, Who Dies: Medical Miracle and a Moral Burden of a Small Committee," *Life*, Nov. 9, 1962, p. 102.

Alvarez, Walter C., "Should We Keep Treating Strenuously an Old Person Who Is Dying?" *Modern Medicine*, Aug. 5, 1969, pp. 73–74.

"An Act of Desperation," *Time*, Vol. 93, April 18, 1969, p. 58.

Anderson, Fred, "Death and Doctors," *The New Republic*, April 19, 1969, pp. 9–10.

Appel, James Z., "Ethical and Legal Questions Posed by Recent Advances in Medicine," *JAMA*, Vol. 205, No. 7 (Aug. 12, 1968), pp. 513–516.

Arnold, John; Zimmerman, Thomas F.; and Martin, Daniel C., "Public Attitudes and the Diagnosis of Death," *JAMA,* Vol. 206, No. 9 (Nov. 25, 1968), pp. 1949–1954.

"Artificial Heart Raises Issues About Ethics," *Medical Tribune,* Vol. 10, April 21, 1969, pp. 1, 21–22.

"Artificial Lung Ready for Patients," *Medical World News,* Vol. 10, Feb. 28, 1969, p. 21.

Barton, R. T., "Sources of Medical Morals," *JAMA,* Vol. 193 (1965), p. 133.

"Baylor Sends Secret Letter in 'Plastic Heart Affair,'" *Medical World News,* Vol. 10, No. 20 (May 16, 1969).

Bean, William B., "On Death," *Arch. Intern. Med.,* Feb., 1958, pp. 199–202.

—— "A Testament of Duty: Some Strictures on Moral Responsibilities in Clinical Research," *J. Lab. Clin. Med.,* Vol. 39 (1952), p. 3.

Beecher, H. K., "Ethics and Clinical Research," *New Eng. J. Med.,* Vol. 274 (1966), p. 1354.

—— "Experimentation in Man," *JAMA,* Vol. 169, Jan. 31, 1959, pp. 461–478.

—— "Some Fallacies and Errors in the Application of the Principle of Consent in Human Experimentation," *Clin. Pharmacol. Ther.,* Vol. 3 (1962), p. 141.

Biorck, G., "Life and Death," *Wisconsin Law Rev.,* Vol. 2 (1968), pp. 484–497.

Brandon, J. M., *et al.,* "Prolongation of Survival by Periodic Prolonged Hemodialysis in Patients with Chronic Renal Failure," *Amer. J. Med.,* Vol. 33 (1962), p. 538.

"British Heart Transplants Stir Up a Storm," *Medical Tribune,* Vol. 10, July 7, 1969, pp. 1, 26.

Buck, R. W., "A Matter of Ethics," *New Eng. J. Med.,* Vol. 274 (1966), p. 1508.

"Cadavers Called Transplant Need," *AMA News,* Vol. 12, March 10, 1969, pp. 1 f.

Cassels, Derek, "UK Transplant Registry Plan Brings

Furious Clash on Ethics," *Medical Post,* Vol. 5, Aug. 12, 1969, p. 1.

——— "Less Support for Heart Transplants, Say Surgeons," *Medical Post,* Vol. 5, Nov. 4, 1969, pp. 11–12.

——— "Heart Donors Volunteer, Says Shumway," *Medical Post,* Vol. 4, Dec. 31, 1968, p. 7.

Chan, E., "Limits for Experimentation," *N.Y.U. Law Rev.,* Vol. 36 (1961), p. 1.

"Chamber Brings Hearts Back Alive," *Medical World News,* Dec. 6, 1968, pp. 25–26.

Collins, Vincent J., "Limits of Medical Responsibility in Prolonging Life," *JAMA,* Vol. 206, No. 2 (Oct. 7, 1968), pp. 389–392.

Connell, F. J., "The Morality of a Kidney Transplantation," *Amer. Eccl. Rev.,* Vol. 138, March, 1958, pp. 205–207.

"Consent in Clinical Experimentation: Myth and Reality," editorial, *JAMA,* Vol. 195 (March 28, 1966), p. 124.

Cooley, Denton A., *et al.,* "Transplantation of the Human Heart," *JAMA,* Vol. 205, No. 7 (Aug. 12, 1968), pp. 479–486.

Curran, William J., "The Law and Human Experimentation," *New Eng. J. Med.,* Vol. 275, No. 6 (Aug. 11, 1966), pp. 323–325.

DeBakey, Michael E., "What's Ahead?" *Medical World News,* March 21, 1969.

Dukeminier, Jesse, Jr., and Sanders, David, "Organ Transplantation: A Proposal for Routine Salvaging of Cadaver Organs," *New Eng. J. Med.,* Vol. 279, No. 8 (Aug. 22, 1968), pp. 413–420.

Elkington, Russell J., "The Changing Mores of Biomedical Research," *Ann. Intern. Med.,* Vol. 67, No. 3, Part 2, Supplement 7 (September, 1967), pp. 3–83.

——— "Medicine and the Quality of Life," *Ann. Intern. Med.,* Vol. 64, No. 3 (March, 1966), pp. 711–714.

——— "Moral Problems in the Use of Borrowed Organs,

Artificial and Transplanted," editorial, *Ann. Intern. Med.*, Vol. 60 (1964), p. 309.

"Ethics of Human Experimentation," editorial, *Brit. Med. J.*, Vol. 2 (July 18, 1964), p. 135.

"Ethics of Medical Progress: Whose Responsibility?" *Hospital Practice*, Dec., 1968, pp. 16–17.

Fishbein, Morris, "Renal Transplantations," *Medical World News*, June 20, 1969, p. 56.

Fletcher, George P., "Legal Aspects of the Decision Not to Prolong Life," *JAMA*, Vol. 203, No. 1 (Jan. 1, 1968), pp. 65–68.

Fletcher, Joseph, "The Patient's Right to Die," *Harper's Magazine*, Oct., 1960, p. 139.

Ford, Thomas J., "Human Organ Transplantations: Legal Aspects," *The Catholic Lawyer*, Vol. 15, No. 2 (Spring, 1969), pp. 136–142, 168.

"42 Per Cent 1-Year Survival Reported for Cadaver Kidneys," *Medical Tribune*, Vol. 10, Aug. 21, 1969, pp. 1, 26–27.

Fox, R. C., "Some Social and Cultural Factors in American Society Conducive to Medical Research on Human Subjects," *Clin. Pharmacol. Ther.*, Vol. 1 (1960), p. 423.

Freund, Paul A., "Ethical Problems in Human Experimentation," *New Eng. J. Med.*, Vol. 273, No. 13 (Sept. 16, 1965), p. 687.

Friedman, George A., "The Lay of the Law," *Medical Opinion and Review*, Vol. 5, No. 2 (Feb., 1969), pp. 15–24.

Frye, William W., "The National Transplant Information Center," *Medical Tribune*, Vol. 10 (Nov. 17, 1969), pp. 19 f.

Giuseppe, B. M.; DeSenarciens, J.; and Groen, J. J., "Human Experimentation—A World Problem from the Standpoint of Spiritual Leaders," *World Med. J.*, Vol. 7 (1960), p. 80.

Halley, Martin M., and Harvey, William F., "Medical vs.

Legal Definitions of Death," *JAMA*, Vol. 204, No. 6 (May 6, 1968), pp. 423–425.

Harken, Dwight Emary, "Transplantation," *JAMA*, Vol. 206, No. 11 (Dec. 9, 1968), p. 2514.

"A Heartbeat Away from the Assembly Line," *Business Week*, Vol. 69, June 14, 1969, p. 130.

Hill, Thomas, "Cooley Explains His Decision to Implant Artificial Heart," *Medical Post*, Vol. 5, May 6, 1969, pp. 2 ff.

"Indiana's Dr. Shumacker, 'Artificial Heart Is . . . Only Ultimate Answer,'" *JAMA*, Vol. 206, No. 6 (Nov. 4, 1968), p. 1197.

Kidd, A. M., "Limits of the Right of a Person to Consent to Experimentation on Himself," *Science*, Vol. 117 (1953), p. 211.

Kretchmar, L. H., *et al.*, "Repeated Hemodialysis in Chronic Uremia," *JAMA*, Vol. 184, No. 13 (June 29, 1963), p. 1030.

Ladimer, I., "Ethical and Legal Aspects of Medical Research on Human Beings," *J. Public Law*, Vol. 3 (1955), p. 467.

———— "Human Experimentation: Medicolegal Aspects," *New Eng. J. Med.*, Vol. 257 (July 4, 1957), pp. 18–24.

Laforet, Eugene G., "The 'Hopeless' Case," *Arch. Intern. Med.*, Vol. 112, Sept., 1963, pp. 314–326.

Lewis, Howard P., "Machine Medicine and Its Relation to the Fatally Ill," *JAMA*, Vol. 206, No. 2 (Oct. 7, 1968), pp. 387–388.

Long, P. H., "On the Quantity and Quality of Life: I. Fruitless Longevity," *Resident Physician*, Vol. 6 (April, 1960), pp. 69–70.

———— "On the Quantity and Quality of Life: II. Moral, Religious, National, and Legal Responsibilities of Physicians in the Care of the Incurably Ill or the Dying," *Resident Physician*, Vol. 6, May, 1960, pp. 53–61.

———— "On the Quantity and Quality of Life: III. A Discussion of the Prolongation of Life in the Incurably Ill and Dying," *Resident Physician,* Vol. 6, June, 1960, pp. 51–53.

McKneally, M., *et al.,* "Procurement of Cadaver Organs for Transplantation," *Surgery,* Vol. 59 (1966), p. 770.

McNeur, Ronald W., "Churches Unite to Explore Questions of Medical Ethics," *Presbyterian Life,* Vol. 22, No. 14 (July 15, 1969), pp. 22–24.

Merrill, John P., "Clinical Experience Is Tempered by Genuine Human Concern," *JAMA,* Vol. 189, No. 8 (Aug. 24, 1964), pp. 626–627.

—— *et al.,* "Successful Homotransplantation of Human Kidney Between Identical Twins," *JAMA,* Vol. 160 (1956), p. 227.

—— "Successful Homotransplantation of Human Kidney Between Nonidentical Twins," *New Eng. J. Med.,* Vol. 262 (1960), p. 1251.

Middleton, John, "Coming: Better Protection for Transplant Teams," *Hospital Physician,* Dec., 1968, pp. 37–44.

Moore, Francis D., *et al.,* "Cardiac and Other Organ Transplantation," *JAMA,* Vol. 206, No. 11 (Dec. 9, 1968), pp. 2489–2500.

—— "Ethics in the New Medicine—Tissue Transplants," *The Nation,* April 5, 1965.

—— "Medical Responsibility for the Prolongation of Life," *JAMA,* Vol. 206, No. 2 (Oct. 7, 1968), pp. 384–386.

Mortimer, R. C., "Moral Issues in Medicine," *Brit. Med. J.,* Vol. 2, July 9, 1960, pp. 128–129.

Murray, J. E., "Human Kidney Transplant Conference," *Transplantation,* Vol. 2 (1964), p. 149.

—— "Proceedings of Conference on Human Kidney Transplants," *Transplantation,* Vol. 2, Jan., 1964, p. 147.

—— Gleason, R., and Bartholomay, A., "Fourth Report of the Human Kidney Transplant Registry: 16 Sept. 1964 to 15 March 1965," *Transplantation,* Vol. 3 (1965), p. 684.

"New Artificial Kidneys," *JAMA*, Vol. 209, Sept. 1, 1969, pp. 1292–1293, 1298.

"New Hearts for Old," *The Herder Correspondence*, Vol. 5, No. 8 (Aug., 1968), pp. 237–242.

"New Power for the Heart," *Business Week*, Vol. 69, June 21, 1969, pp. 104, 106.

"New Probes in Plastic Heart Affair," *Medical World News*, Vol. 10, June 13, 1969, p. 22.

"Nuclear-powered Pacer 'Should Run 20 Years,'" *Medical Tribune*, Vol. 10, June 26, 1969, pp. 1, 20.

"Organ Transplants," panel discussion, American Association of Railway Surgeons, *Industrial Medicine and Surgery*, Vol. 38, Dec., 1969, pp. 415–422.

Page, Irvine H., "The Ethics of Heart Transplantation," *JAMA*, Vol. 207, No. 1 (Jan. 6, 1969), pp. 109–113.

———— "Unwise Publicity," editorial, *Modern Medicine*, Jan. 27, 1964, p. 81.

———— "Prolongation of Life in Affluent Society," editorial, *Modern Medicine*, Oct. 14, 1963, p. 89.

———— "What Strange Values," *Modern Medicine*, Nov. 4, 1968, p. 65.

Platt, R., "Reflections on Medicine and Humanism," Progress Report to Thomas Linacre, Linacre Lecture, 1963, *University Quarterly*, Vol. 17 (1963), p. 327.

"Prolongation of Dying," editorial, *Lancet*, Vol. 2 (1962), p. 1205.

Reemtsma, K., *et al.*, "Renal Heterotransplantation in Man," *Ann. Surg.*, Vol. 160 (1964), p. 384.

Retan, J. W., and Lewis, H. Y., "Repeated Dialysis of Indigent Patients in Chronic Renal Failure," *Ann. Intern. Med.*, Vol. 64 (1966), p. 284.

Rhoads, Paul S., "Medical Ethics and Morals in a New Age," *JAMA*, Vol. 205, No. 7 (Aug. 12, 1968), pp. 517–522.

Riley, C. M., "Thoughts About Kidney Homotransplantation in Children," *J. Pediat.*, Vol. 65 (1964), p. 797.

Robberts, C., "The Modern Biologist and Humanism," *Perspect. Biol. Med.*, Vol. 6 (1963), p. 188.

Robin, E. D., "Rapid Advances Bring New Ethical Questions: Transplantation and Morality," *JAMA*, Vol. 189 (Aug. 24, 1964), p. 112.

"Rushing Donor Organs," *Medical World News*, July 18, 1969, pp. 28–34.

Sadler, Alfred M., *et al.*, "Transplantation—A Case for Consent," *New Eng. J. Med.*, Vol. 280, No. 16 (April 17, 1969), pp. 862–868.

———— "The Uniform Anatomical Gift Act," *JAMA*, Vol. 206, No. 11 (Dec. 9, 1968), pp. 2501–2506.

Schreiner, G. E., and Maher, J. F., "Hemodialysis for Chronic Renal Failure. III. Medical, Moral and Ethical, and Socio-Economic Problems," *Ann. Intern. Med.*, Vol. 62 (1965), p. 551.

Scribner, B. H., "Ethical Problems of Using Artificial Organs to Sustain Human Life," *Trans. Amer. Soc. Artif. Intern. Organs*, Vol. 10 (1964), p. 209.

———— *et al.*, "The Treatment of Chronic Uremia by Means of Intermittent Hemodialysis," *Trans. Amer. Soc. Artif. Intern. Organs*, Vol. 6 (1960), p. 114.

Segal, Charles N., "Medical Malpractice in an Organ Transplant Case," *Trial Lawyers Quarterly*, Vol. 6, No. 2 (Spring/Summer, 1969), pp. 47–53.

Starzl, T. E., *et al.*, "The Role of Organ Transplantation in Pediatrics," *Pediat. Clin. N. Amer.*, Vol. 13 (1966), p. 381.

"Statement on Heart Transplantation," *JAMA*, Vol. 207, No. 9 (March 3, 1969), pp. 1704–1705.

Stevens, Leonard A., "When Is Death?" *Reader's Digest*, Vol. 94, No. 565 (May, 1969), pp. 225–232.

Stickel, D. L., *et al.*, "Renal Transplantation with Donor-Recipient Tissue-Matching: Preliminary Report of First Case in North Carolina," *N. Carolina Med. J.*, Vol. 26 (1965), p. 379.

Stumpf, S. E., "Some Moral Dimensions of Medicine,"
    Ann. Intern. Med., Vol. 64 (1966), p. 460.
Taussig, Helen B., "A Time for Waiting," *The Johns Hop-
    kins Magazine*, Spring, 1969, pp. 9–11.
"Too Much, Too Fast?" *Newsweek*, Vol. 73, April 21, 1969,
    pp. 76, 78.
"Transplant Caucus Balks at Backing Mondale Bill,"
    JAMA, Vol. 206, No. 3 (Oct. 14, 1968), pp. 492–493.
"Transplant Psychosis," *Newsweek*, Vol. 73, May 19, 1969,
    p. 118.
Transplantation, editorial, Vol. 4 (1966), p. 237.
"Transplanters' New Hope: Anticoagulants," *Medical
    World News*, June 27, 1969, pp. 14–15.
"Transplants: Guarded Outlook," *Newsweek*, July 21,
    1969, pp. 109–110.
"Uniform Anatomical Gift Act Aimed at Interstate Bar-
    riers," *JAMA*, Vol. 206, No. 3 (Oct. 14, 1968), pp.
    493–494.
Vaux, Kenneth, "A Year of Heart Transplants: An Ethical
    Evaluation," *Postgraduate Medicine*, Jan., 1969, pp.
    201–205.
Veith, Ilza, and Zimmerman, Lee M., "Further Reflec-
    tions on Organ Transplants," *Modern Medicine*, Oct. 7,
    1968, pp. 153–158.
Wasmuth, Carl E., "Law and Medicine," *Medical World
    News*, Jan. 17, 1969, p. 75.
——— "The Physician's Role in Organ Transplantation,"
    Modern Medicine, June 30, 1969, p. 70.
Weisman, A. D., and Hackett, T. P., "Predilection to
    Death: Death and Dying as a Psychiatric Problem,"
    Psychosomatic Med., Vol. 23 (May–June, 1961), pp.
    232–236.
Welt, L. G., "Reflections on the Problems of Human
    Experimentation," *Conn. Med.*, Vol. 25 (1961), p. 75.
"What and When Is Death?" *JAMA*, Vol. 204, No. 6
    (May 6, 1968), pp. 219–220.
"What Does a New Heart Do to the Mind?" *Medical

World News, May 23, 1969, pp. 17–18.

"When Do You Pull the Plug?" *JAMA,* Vol. 205, No. 1 (July 1, 1968), pp. 29–30.

Woodruff, M. F. A., "Ethical Problems in Organ Transplantation," *Brit. Med. J.,* Vol. 1, June 6, 1964, pp. 1457–1460.

World Medical Association, "Draft Code of Ethics on Human Experimentation," *Brit. Med. J.,* Vol. 2 (1962), p. 1119.

NEWSPAPERS

AMA News, March 31, 1969.

Chicago's American, April 6, 7, 1969.

Chicago Daily News, April 5, 7, 8, 1969.

Chicago Sun-Times, Dec. 7, 1968; April 5, 1969; Sept. 7, 1969.

Chicago Today, May 1, 1969.

Chicago Tribune, April 8, 1969.

New York Times, Feb. 21, 1969; April 11, 1969; July 18, 1969; Aug. 19, 1969.

Pittsburgh Press, Nov. 29, 30, 1968; Dec. 6, 13, 1968; April 5, 9, 1969.

Pittsburgh Post-Gazette, Dec. 9, 12, 16, 20, 1968; April 5, 9, 1969.

This Week, Nov. 17, 1968; June 22, 1969.

U.S. Medicine, Nov. 1, 15, 1968; April 15, 1969.

Wall Street Journal, April 7, 17, 1969; July 17, 1969; Oct. 16, 1969.

UNPUBLISHED MATERIALS

Ayd, Frank J., "What Is Death?" Unpublished article presented at the Second National Congress on Medical Ethics, sponsored by the Judicial Council of the American Medical Association, Chicago, Ill., Oct. 5–6, 1968. (Xeroxed.)

Kolbe, Henry E., "The Permission of Death: A Question in Ethics and Medicine." Unpublished article presented to The American Society of Christian Ethics at Wesley Theological Seminary, Washington, D.C., Jan. 23, 1965. (Xeroxed.)

Surgery Training Committee of the National Institutes of Health, "Status of Transplantation 1968." Unpublished report, Bethesda, Md., Nov., 1968. (Mimeographed.)